The Managen of Pain in Older People

Edited by

PAT SCHOFIELD, PHD RGN

BICENTENNIAL
1807
WILEY
2007
BICENTENNIAL

John Wiley & Sons, Ltd

Copyright © 2007   John Wiley & Sons Ltd
                          The Atrium, Southern Gate, Chichester,
                          West Sussex PO19 8SQ, England
                          Telephone   (+44) 1243 779777

Email (for orders and customer service enquiries): cs-books@wiley.co.uk
Visit our Home Page on www.wiley.com

Other Wiley Editorial Offices

John Wiley & Sons Inc., 111 River Street, Hoboken, NJ 07030, USA

Jossey-Bass, 989 Market Street, San Francisco, CA 94103-1741, USA

Wiley-VCH Verlag GmbH, Boschstr. 12, D-69469 Weinheim, Germany

John Wiley & Sons Australia Ltd, 42 McDougall Street, Milton, Queensland 4064, Australia

John Wiley & Sons (Asia) Pte Ltd, 2 Clementi Loop #02-01, Jin Xing Distripark, Singapore 129809

John Wiley & Sons Canada Ltd, 6045 Freemont Blvd, Mississauga, ONT, L5R 4J3.

Wiley also publishes its books in a variety of electronic formats. Some content that appears in print may
not be available in electronic books.

Anniversary Logo Design: Richard J. Pacifico

Library of Congress Cataloging-in-Publication Data

The management of pain in older people / edited by Pat Schofield.
        p.   ;   cm.
   Includes bibliographical references.
   ISBN 978-0-470-03349-4 (pbk. : alk. paper)
1. Pain in old age.   I. Schofield, Pat (Patricia A.)
   [DNLM: 1. Pain – therapy.   2. Age Factors.   3. Aged.   4. Aging – physiology.
WL 704 M26635 2007]
   RB127.M365 2007
   616'.0472 – dc22
                                                            2006100400

A catalogue record for this book is available from the British Library

ISBN 978-0-470-03349-4

Printed and bound in Great Britain by TJ International Ltd, Padstow, Cornwall

This book is printed on acid-free paper responsibly manufactured from sustainable forestry in which at
least two trees are planted for each one used for paper production.

The Management of Pain in
Older People

Contents

Contributors

Barry Aveyard BA (Hons) MA CertEd RMN RGN RNT

Barry is qualified in both adult and mental health nursing. His experience covers a wide range of clinical settings, but working with older people is his key area of interest. He has worked in nurse education for several years as a teacher and lecturer, and is also a member of the RCN Mental Health and Older Peoples Nursing Forum. Barry has published a number of book chapters and research papers on varying aspects of older people's mental health.

Amanda Clarke BA (Hons) MA PhD RGN

Amanda is a lecturer in the School of Nursing and Midwifery at the University of Sheffield. She completed her nurse training at Sheffield in 1986 and subsequently specialized in the care of older adults. During her nursing career, Amanda worked as a staff nurse and senior sister in stroke rehabilitation and acute medicine for older people. As a mature student, she undertook her undergraduate and post-graduate degrees in the Department of Sociological Studies at the University of Sheffield. She gained her BA in Social and Political Studies in 1994 and her MA in Applied Research and Quality Evaluation in 1996. In 2001, Amanda completed her doctorate exploring older people's accounts of their experiences and attitudes to later life, using a biographical approach. She also worked as a research associate on the European Funded project ACTION (Assisting Carers Using Telematic Interventions to Meet Older Person's Needs). Her research interests include life story work with older people, participatory ways of working with older people, active ageing, and end-of-life care in later life.

Mary Cooke BSc(Hons) MSc(Econs) PGCert PhD RGN CertMld

Mary has a clinical background in surgical nursing and midwifery, where she has held posts as clinical sister and manager and as assistant to a chief nurse. She still practices in accident and emergency care. Her academic career began in 1984 while she was a staff nurse, and progressed with a masters in planning and financing health care at the London School of Economics while working in higher education, followed by a PhD from the same institution. She has held consultant research roles and was a research associate while completing postdoctoral studies at the University of Cambridge. Mary is now a lecturer at Sheffield Hallam University, seconded to the University of Sheffield, and specializes in health policy, health economics and service user involvement.

Rachel Drago RN MSc PGDipEd DipTher

Rachel is a lecturer in nursing at the University of the West of England, Bristol. She has staffed in hospitals in London, Leeds and Nottingham and worked as a lecturer in nursing since 1995, specializing in the teaching of physiology whilst working as a critical care practitioner. Rachel now teaches human physiology, functional anatomy and clinical pharmacology to nurses at all levels of study.

Margaret Dunham BA(Hons) MSc RGN

Margaret has over five years' experience of clinical practice in pain management and has maintained links with current pain management practice through her membership of the British Pain Society, Pain Network UK and the North Trent Pain Forum. She is on the national committee of Pain Network UK, supporting nurses in practice throughout the UK and Ireland. Since leaving the NHS in 2000 to lecture at the University of Sheffield Margaret has collaborated in the development of educational strategies to promote the needs of older people in pain. She has presented poster abstracts of her work at national and international conferences and is currently building a portfolio of publications. She currently lectures in nursing and pain management at Sheffield Hallam University.

Denis Martin BSc (Hons) MSc DPhil

Denis is a reader in rehabilitation in the Teesside Centre for Rehabilitation Sciences at Teesside University. He previously worked as a principal research fellow in the Centre for Health and Social Care Research at Sheffield Hallam University and was a director of the Scottish Network for Chronic Pain Research and award coordinator of the MSc Pain at Queen Margaret University College, Edinburgh. He graduated from the University of Ulster in 1988 with a BSc (Hons) in physiotherapy, was awarded his DPhil from the University of Ulster in 1993 and received an MSc in applied statistics from Napier University in 2000. He is a member of the International Association for the Study of Pain, the Pain Society and the Royal Statistical Society. His research interests lie in the assessment and management of the impact of pain. He has published widely in the field of pain. Denis is Chair of the Pain Association, a not-for-profit organization that provides training and support in the self-management of chronic pain.

David Reid BA(Hons) MSc

David is currently a lecturer at the School of Nursing and Midwifery, University of Sheffield. He has previously worked for the Alzheimer's Society, providing support to people with dementia and their carers and coordinating the development of a new branch of the organization in East Yorkshire. David has also previously been a research fellow, when he contributed to qualitative and quantitative studies in the areas of hospice-based adult bereavement support, end-of-life care, partnership and inclusion practices of the Alzheimer's Society in Yorkshire and adult protection. David has published a number of journal articles and has a particular interest in the ways in which the identities of people with dementia are negotiated in social interaction.

Tony Ryan BSc (Hons) MA PhD

Tony is currently a senior lecturer in the Faculty of Health and Wellbeing at Sheffield Hallam University. For almost eight years he worked with people with learning difficulties in a research and development capacity. Following a move to the University of Sheffield, he became involved in work with people with dementia. Tony was instrumental in local service developments, most significantly in the initiation and expansion of community-based provision. He worked within the Institute of General Practice and Primary Care where he completed his PhD (2003), before moving to the School of Nursing and Midwifery in 2004. In 2006 he joined Sheffield Hallam University, where he teaches on a range of programmes. His research interests centre on people with dementia and their family carers as well as stroke and pain for older people

Pat Schofield PGDipEd DipN PhD RGN

Pat has worked in the field of pain management since 1989, first as a clinical nurse specialist and for the last ten years as a lecturer and now as a senior lecturer in the School of Nursing and Midwifery at the University of Sheffield. She was originally responsible for the development of the pain modules and is currently the unit leader to the acute, chronic and age-related units. Pat's research involves the use of Snoezelen environments for the management of chronic pain and palliative care. More recently, she has completed a study looking at resident's perceptions of pain in care homes and a systematic review of the literature in the first stage of a funded project to investigate pain in this setting within the UK. Pat has recently developed a distance learning pain education package for staff caring for older adults in care homes, being introduced around the UK in collaboration with the English Care in the Community Association.

Paula Smith BSc (Hons) MSc PhD DEN RN C.Psychol

Paula is a lecturer and programme leader for the MMedSci in Palliative Care at the School of Nursing and Midwifery, University of Sheffield She has a background in Community Nursing and Health Psychology. In 2001 Paula completed her PhD which focused on the support needs of family caregivers in palliative care settings in the community. Since then she has worked on a number of research projects, primarily in community palliative care settings, and has interests in family caregivers, service development and evaluation. Paula is currently a steering group member of Help the Hospices Care for the Carers of the Terminally Ill Project.

The anatomy and physiology of pain

1

Pat Schofield and Rachel Drago

The human body is able to experience a range of sensations, from the pleasant, soothing texture of velvet to the extremely unpleasant sensation of pain. For many years it has been acknowledged that the process of pain does not consist solely of a physiological set of sensations: it is a combination of physiological sensations that requires complex physiological, psychological and behavioural interactions to enable the human to interpret and subsequently respond (Wall and Melzack, 1999).

The aims of this chapter are:

- To discuss the concepts underpinning the physiology of pain.
- To explore the gate control theory of pain.
- To highlight the changes that occur within the nervous system as a result of ageing that may impact upon the pain experience as the person ages.
- To demonstrate how an understanding of these factors may influence practice.

Generally, everyone perceives the pain experience to be unpleasant and to be avoided at all costs. Only a few reported individuals are known to have never experienced pain, and this is now a recognized syndrome (hereditary sensory and autonomic neuropathy type 4). Pain is wholly subjective, and the perceived intensity and discomfort for any one known controlled stimulus varies from person to person. The actual perception of pain requires a complicated integration of sensory nerves, motor nerve pathways and chemicals that serve to enhance the pain. All of these can be influenced by the genetic make-up of the individual, their past experiences and emotional contributors. This means that the sensation of pain is greater that the sum of its parts.

Although pain pathways, physiology and local hormone production play only a small part in the overall sensation of pain, the efficacy of analgesics and other pharmacological therapies is based on the modulation of the nervous system and its role in the sensation of pain. It is essential for any health-care professional to have good understanding of the anatomy and physiology of pain in order to make informed decisions regarding the most appropriate therapy.

Learning point

Revise some of the following terminology:

- peripheral and central nervous system
- spinal cord
- sensory cortex
- simple spinal reflex
- synapse, neurotransmitters and receptors
- sensory afferents
- motor and autonomic efferent
- autonomic nervous system.

You may wish to read the paper by Davis (1993) and the book by Melzack and Wall (1996) to support your learning.

Pain and sensation

The definition of pain as

an unpleasant sensory or emotional experience associated with actual or potential tissue damage or described in terms of such damage (Merskey and Bogduk 1992, p. 210) suggests that pain may be the result of actual or potential tissue damage and that it prevents the individual from bodily harm, or from the injury, disease or harm becoming worse. It is a dramatic mixture of emotional and physiological reactions (Mountcastle, 1980; Merskey, 1986; Wall and Melzack, 1999).

There are certain things that we now know to occur within the nervous system when a disease or injury arises, but there are still some things we don't know about. Research into these mechanisms is ongoing. In this section we discuss the basic physiological concepts and then we consider the issues that are particularly relevant for the care of older people.

Imagine putting your hand on to a hot stove. This will initiate a series of responses within the nervous system that will eventually be perceived as pain. The whole process begins at the site of the injury, or 'where your hand is touching the hot stove'.

Physiological pain arises from chemical, thermal or mechanical stimulus of the small-diameter sensory afferent fibres found in the tissue. These actually detect injury and are known as **nociceptors**, which derives from the Latin word meaning injury. It is important to be aware of this as it helps us to understand the concepts of **neuropathic** and **nociceptive** pain.

Learning point

Can you identify the differences between neuropathic and nociceptive pain?
Think about the types of neuropathic pain that you see in your area.

There are two types of nociceptors: **Aδ** (A delta) and **C fibres** (Cesare and McNaughton, 1997). These are different from other sensory afferent nerve fibres in that the noxious stimulus has to be of a sufficient intensity and duration to bring about tissue damage. In other words, these fibres have a high stimulation threshold. Tactile fibres such as **Aβ** (A beta) fibres have a low threshold and follow slightly different spinal tracts to the brain. They also transfer information related to pressure and texture, but not pain. To illustrate this, imagine what it would be like if pain was initiated by a soft touch – such inappropriate misfiring would make life impossible. Equally, if the nociceptors' threshold is set too high then tissue damage would result before avoidance action could be taken. Hence the stimulation intensity is set to prevent unnecessary tissue damage or discomfort.

Modulation and regulation of all of the incoming information is carried out by nerves that descend from the brain to the spinal cord and contribute to the analysis of the sensations at this level. These **descending tracts** are responsible for the regulation of sensations that actually reach the brain and allow the individual to divert their attention elsewhere. This is the rudimentary basis of the **gate control theory** which we will return to later.

We can consider two categories of pain:

- **Physiological pain:** The pain response to high-intensity stimuli is transient if the tissue damage is prevented by a simple spinal flexion reflex arc (Willer, 1979). Consider striking a match and touching the flame with your fingers – you would drop the match instantly before damage could occur. The speed with which this reflex occurs prevents deep tissue damage and allows only a brief moment of discomfort. This is caused by a simple spinal reflex mediated by the high-intensity thermal stimulation of small sensory nerve endings in your fingers.

- **Pathological pain:** This results from sensitization of the nerves in the periphery and the spinal cord. Peripheral nerve endings are made more sensitive to noxious stimuli through tissue damage, action of local hormones such as prostaglandins, histamine, serotonin and bradykinin, and also by direct nerve damage – this is called **peripheral sensitization**.

When the **neurons** involved with the transmission of pain along the spinal cord to the sensory cortex in the parietal lobe of the brain are sensitized by a barrage of impulses from the site of tissue damage, this is referred to as **central sensitization**. As a result the nerve fibres of the central nervous system begin to respond to non-noxious stimuli such as gentle touch as if they were pain impulses. Peripheral and central sensitization of the neural pathway can produce pain without a clear external stimulus. So, for example, gentle stroking can become pain – this is termed **allodynia**. Furthermore, an exaggerated response to low-threshold noxious stimuli can occur (**hyperalgesia**) (Woolf, 1989, 1991; Rang, Dale and Ritter, 1999). In acute pain, this is quite an important concept as potentiation of pain will encourage rest and thus prevent further tissue damage (Woolf, 1991). However, should this continue after the acute phase (i.e. in **chronic pain**) it will serve no useful purpose and become a clinical problem in its own right. This will be discussed later, in Chapter 6.

Summary

- Pain is an unpleasant sensation which warns of impending tissue damage.
- Pain develops as a results of chemical, thermal or mechanical stimuli.
- Activation of A-δ and C fibres occurs; these are known as nociceptors and they detect injury, not pain.

- A-β fibres transmit pressure, not pain.
- The physiological response to high-intensity is transient if the tissue damage is prevented by a simple spinal flexion reflex arc.
- Sensitization of nerves in the periphery and spinal cord is known as pathological pain.
- Tissue damage or local hormone action can make peripheral nerve endings more sensitive this is known as peripheral sensitization.
- When the central nervous system responds to Aβ fibres as if they were conducting pain impulses, central sensitization occurs.

Neural pain pathways

When the sensory neurons synapse with the motor neurons and transmission neurons in the dorsal horn of the spinal cord, pain is detected. As seen in Figure 1.1, the nerve fibres within the dorsal horn (rear) carry information back to the spinal cord and brain. The ventral horn (front) carries autonomic efferents and motor nerves away from the spinal cord and brain back to the body.

The terminal nerve endings of the sensory nociceptors release the neurotransmitters **substance P** and **glutamate**. These chemicals in turn bind to the surface of the dendrites of the transmission neurons, propagating the signal forward either to a motor nerve or up to the brain via the spinal cord.

C fibres

These are fine **unmyelinated fibres**, 0.23–1.5 μm in diameter, which respond to chemical, thermal or mechanical stimuli. Because they have more than one mode

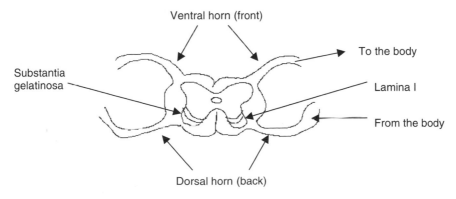

Figure 1.1 Cross-section of the spinal cord

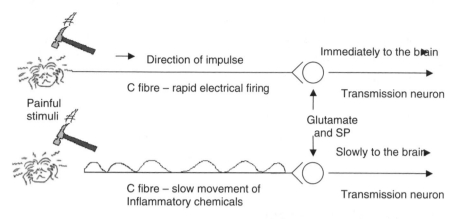

Figure 1.2   The rapid and slow effects of the C fibre in the dorsal horn

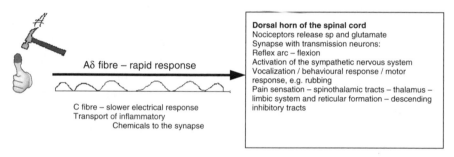

Figure 1.3   Physiological pain responses

of stimulation they are also known as **polymodal fibres**. It is believed that C-fibre activity is associated with dull, diffuse pain and once initiated can continue for up to 80 hours. The conduction velocity (speed with which the pain message travels) is <2.5 m/s (Figure 1.2).

Along with sending electrical messages to the spinal cord by the movement of potassium and sodium ions into and out of the axon, C fibres are also responsible for the absorption of inflammatory chemicals such as **bradykinin** along the length of the axon to be released within the spinal cord at the synapse with the transmission neuron (Wall and Melzack, 1999). This process provides a dull, diffuse and profound ache that often follows relatively minor injuries such as a sprained ankle, resulting in the whole leg aching for days after the injury.

Aδ fibres

These are medium-sized (1–5 μm diameter), myelinated, fast-acting neurons with a rapid conduction velocity (>2 m/s) (Figure 1.3). It is believed that these neurons are responsible for the sensation of well-localized, sharp and intense pain (Rang, Dale and Ritter, 1999). The function of Aδ fibres is similar to that of C fibres, but they react more rapidly and are sensitive to thermal and mechanical stimuli only.

Think of how it feels when you prick yourself with a needle. Initially you feel the exact point of the pain. But a few minutes later, the pain became more widespread and it becomes difficult to locate the exact site of the injury. What we are feeling is the initial Aδ pain followed by the C fibre pain. Both Aδ and C fibres are found in large numbers in the skin, but C fibres predominate in the internal organs, muscles and viscera. However, both types of fibres set up a reaction that moves along the axons to the synapse with a number of transmission neurons within the dorsal horn of the spinal cord and along tracts to the brain.

At the site of injury we have a group of nerve fibres that will begin the process.

Learning point

Can you complete the table below?

Nerve fibre	Myelin sheath	Type of sensation
Aδ	?	?
C	?	Dull aching
Aβ	Yes	?

Dorsal roots

The next stage of the pain processing pathway is the spinal cord. Both Aδ and C fibres enter the spinal cord at the **dorsal horn**. The dorsal roots are made of layers, known as **laminae**, into which the sensory nerve fibres enter. Synapses are made with the transmission neurons that direct the impulse across the spinal cord to motor neurons and can elicit a reflex flexion arc from the offending source of the noxious stimuli. Alternatively, the impulse may ascend the spinal cord to the brain.

Within the spinal cord is a neuron-rich area which is known as the **substantia gelatinosa**. All sensory fibres have to cross this area before forming a synapse with spinal neurons in the various laminae. It is believed that the Aδ and C fibres connect within the layers I–III.

The substantia gelatinosa contains short nerve fibres (**interneurons**) which regulate the transmission of impulses from nociceptors and other sensory nerve fibres. Interneurons are rich in neurotransmitters which resemble opiates and are therefore very important in the modulation of nociception through an opiate receptor mechanism. These chemicals, known as endorphins, are very similar to morphine.

Learning point

Endorphins are opiates produced naturally by the body.

It may be useful at this point to consider the marathon runner. After running for about 10–15 miles – around half way in the 26-mile race – the runner experiences excruciating pain, but if they continue to run, they pass through what is known as the **pain barrier**. At this point the pain begins to subside, because the person has started to produce the endogenous opioids which act like morphine and control the pain. Although we are all capable of producing these chemicals, most of us tend to ask for drugs instead of relying on our internal mechanisms. It has been suggested that it can take a few days to get these opioids out of the system.

Furthermore, the interneurons inhibit the response of the transmission neurons to stimulation from an Aδ fibre when impulses generated by an Aβ fibre are also arriving at the synapse with the transmission neurons. At a time of high input from nociceptors the large Aβ fibres which respond to pressure and mechanical stimuli are filtered through the substantia gelatinosa in the spinal cord. These Aβ fibres are much larger that the other two types and therefore can transmit their sensations much quicker, thus blocking the pain messages being carried by the other two. The Aβ fibres are activated by rubbing the area.

Learning point

Massage is a pain-relieving techniques that works on this principle.

Spinal cord to brain

As the impulse travels through the various centres within the brain, the sensation of pain is perceived. Furthermore, the sympathetic nervous system is aroused and consequently the individual experiences an increased blood pressure, heart rate and increased blood flow. The organism experiences a heightened sense of arousal or wakefulness. The sympathetic nervous system, which responds to **E situations** (emergency, excitement and embarrassment), dominates the regulation of the body and prepares it for 'fight or flight'. Adrenalin is secreted by the adrenal medulla and noradrenaline is secreted into the injured tissue.

Simultaneously, the individual experiences higher brain centre responses which include vocalization and behavioural responses – oh ****! Arousal and emotional effects occur as a result of increased involvement in other areas of the brain.

The problem is that there is no one centre in the brain that is responsible for pain processing. Therefore almost all of the brain becomes involved, which is why pain is often difficult to treat.

Learning point

Read around the role of the brain and identify the functions of some of the major structures listed below:

Structure	Function
Cortices	
Thalamus	
Limbic system	
Reticular activating system	

The Aδ and C fibres exist throughout the body, on the periphery, viscera and internal organs – with one exception. There is one place where we do not feel pain. Think of Hannibal Lecter! That's right; the internal substance of the brain has no pain receptors. But before you test this theory by putting a hatchet in someone's head, remember that the scalp and the outer coverings of the brain do contain the receptors that enable us to feel pain.

Descending tracts and substantia gelatinosa

Descending tracts are efferent fibres which leave the reticular formation within the brain, travel along the spinal cord and synapse with the transmission and interneurons within the substantia gelatinosa. The descending tracts function in order to modulate incoming messages from peripheral nerves. Thus, they act as a filter and partial inhibitor of the messages ascending the spinal cord from the nociceptors. This limits transmission of the impulses from the sensory Aδ and C fibres along the transmission fibres.

The descending nerve fibres arise at the **periaqueductal grey** within the reticular formation and flow into the **medulla** (brainstem). From the specific area called the **nucleus raphe magnus** in the medulla, impulses then pass down the dorsolateral tracts in the spinal cord to connect with the transmission neurons and interneurons in the substantia gelatinosa of the spinal cord (Fields and Basbaum, 1994). The major neurotransmitter from the descending tracts is **serotonin**, which stimulates interneurons within the substantia gelatinosa to release peptides, noradrenaline and endogenous opioids such as **endorphins**, **enkephalins** and **dynorphines**. All of the areas associated with pain processing are rich in opiate receptors, which could explain the actions of our analgesic preparations. The pain pathway is a cycle of events within the central nervous system, interpreting and modulating the impulses that are generated in the peripheral nerves of the body.

Learning point

Revise the autonomic, peripheral and central nervous systems.

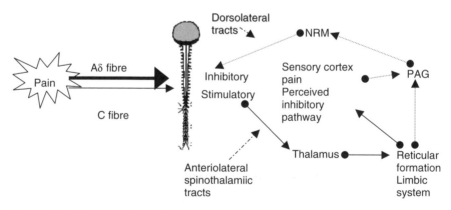

Figure 1.4 The ascending pathways and descending inhibitory pathways. SG, substantia gelatinosa; PAG, periaqueductal grey; NRM, nucleus raphe magnus. Dashed lines show pain modulation pathways (descending); solid lines show pain sensation pathways (ascending)

Summary

- Nociceptors synapse with motor and transmission neurons in the dorsal horn of the spinal cord.
- Transmission fibres within dorsal horn carry information to the brain and spinal cord.
- The dorsal horn is made up of layers (laminae) which contain many transmission neurons.
- Aδ and C fibres synapse with transmission neurons in the first three layers of the spinal cord (laminae I–III).
- Nociceptors release the neurotransmitter (substance P or glutamate).
- The substantia gelatinosa is a neuron-rich area through which all nociceptors pass before forming a synapse with spinal neurons in the various laminae.
- The interneurons within the substantia gelatinosa regulate the transmission of impulses from the nociceptors and other sensory nerve fibres to the various laminae. These are rich in neurotransmitters that resemble opiates and are important in the modulation of nociception through an opiate receptor mechanism.
- C fibres are unmyelinated and respond to chemical, thermal and mechanical stimuli; they precipitate dull, diffuse pain.
- Aδ fibres are myelinated and therefore produce sharp, shooting stabbing pain that is well localized.

The pain gate

The pain gate was proposed by Melzack and Wall back in 1965. It is the most widely accepted theory of pain, and explains a great many of the pain phenomena. But the theory is by no means complete, and work continues to refine it. The **plasticity** of the nervous system – its ability to become desensitized and sensitized – also adds an extra dimension (Figure 1.5).

Aδ and C fibres synapse within the dorsal horn of the spinal cord with both transmission fibres and interneurons. This is true for the Aβ fibres also. Tissue damage produces high-intensity messages which move along the nociceptors to the transmission neuron. The nociceptors also form synapses with small excitatory interneurons. Concurrent stimulation of the excitatory interneuron as well as the transmission neuron will augment the nociceptors' output and hence potentiate the pain experience. Rubbing the affected area will also stimulate the

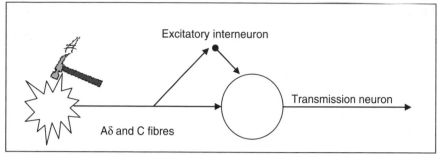

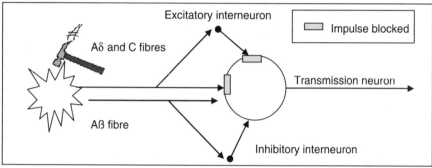

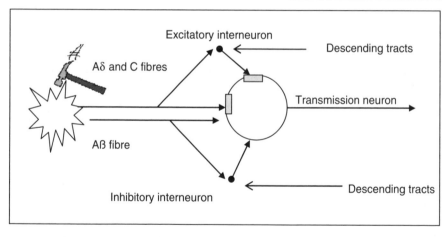

Figure 1.5 A simple pain pathway

low-threshold Aβ fibres which in turn synapse with the **inhibitory interneuron** which decreases sensitivity of the transmission neuron to the nociceptors' outputs. The descending pathways of the periaqueductal grey will attempt to modulate the activity of the interneuron by stimulating the inhibitory interneurons to release endogenous opioids, thus blocking the nociceptive pathway.

Learning point

How does this fit with some of the strategies that we may use for pain control, such as heat or TENS?

Summary

- The gate control theory is the most widely accepted theory of pain sensation and inhibition. It has yet to be disproved, but other theories do exist.

- Plasticity is the ability of the nervous system to become sensitized or desensitized.

- Aδ and C nociceptors and Aβ sensory fibres synapse with the same interneurons.

- Painful stimuli excite the nociceptors, which in turn excite the transmission neuron and excitatory interneurons

- Rubbing the affected area excites Aβ sensory fibres. These synapse with an inhibitory interneuron, which decrease sensitivity of the transmission neuron to the nociceptors outputs.

- The descending tracts modulate the pain sensation by stimulating the inhibitory interneurons to release endogenous opiates, blocking the nociceptive pathway.

For a recent survey of the gate control theory, see the article by Dickenson (2002).

Chronic pain

All of this physiology appears fairly straightforward. But as we can see in Chapter 6, the whole system becomes much more complicated when we discuss chronic pain or pain that appears to have no identifiable physical cause. We are aware that pain sensations travel through many parts of the brain in their journey towards interpretation. This journey could in some way explain the ramifications and issues that arise from chronic pain as the individual becomes increasingly depressed and disillusioned, along with the involvement of the sympathetic nervous system and the inability to find sleep or comfort that is often described by chronic pain sufferers. However, this is not the complete picture. The plasticity of the central nervous system and the change in sensitivity of peripheral nerves and central pathways also adds support to the signs and symptoms reported by patients with chronic pain. Therefore when dealing with chronic pain, we need to look beyond the usual approaches with analgesics and adopt more creative approaches that would not be considered for the management of acute pain.

Peripheral sensitization

When tissues are damaged they cause the release of phospholipids from the plasma cell membrane. Enzymes such as phospholipase A_2 exist in the cell membrane and catalyse the breakdown of phospholipids into arachidonic acid which can be further modified by other enzymes (cycloxygenases 1 and 2 and lipogenase) to produce a family of chemicals known as **eicosanoids**. These are often referred to as **local hormones** and include substances such as prostaglandins, leukotrienes, lipoxins, chemotaxins and thromboxancs. These eicosanoids act on the C fibres and thus increase their sensitivity, which increases the unpleasant experience of pain. The C fibres can also absorb many of these chemicals and pass them along to the dorsal horn via the axons (Figure 1.6).

The nociceptors also release inflammatory mediators into the surrounding tissue, which adds impact to the action of local hormones. Hence when stimulated by high-intensity heat, chemical or mechanical activity, the nociceptors also release **calcitonin gene related peptide** (CGRP) and substance P (Brain and Williams, 1985). These chemicals act directly upon mast cells (connective tissue

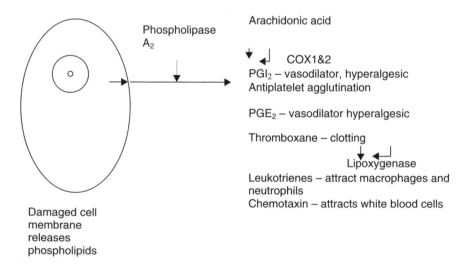

Figure 1.6 Cell damage and arachidonic acid

cells containing granules of histamine), causing the release of histamine and serotonin. Substance P and CGRP also act upon the local blood vessels, causing vasodilatation and increased capillary permeability (Figure 1.7).

The sympathetic nerves in the damaged area add to the cocktail of inflammatory chemicals by releasing prostaglandin I_2 and monoamines such as noradrenaline. The inflammatory cocktail alters the threshold of peripheral nociceptors to increase sensitivity of the neuron. This is done in several ways; by coupling to the receptors on the neuron and opening up ion channels, thus lowering the action potential threshold, or indirectly by increasing the number of ion channels within the nociceptive membrane (Figure 1.8).

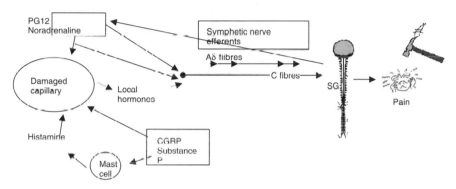

Figure 1.7 Peripheral sensitization by the sympathetic efferents, local hormones and local release of nociceptors derived from substance P

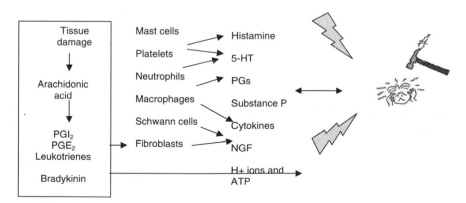

Figure 1.8 The inflammatory chemical cocktail and increased peripheral pain perception

The inflammatory mediation of peripheral sensitization mechanisms explains the anti-inflammatory and analgesic effects of non-steroidal anti-inflammatory drugs (NSAIDs) and glutocorticoids (steroids) which inhibit the lipoxygenase and cycloxygenase enzymes and so reduce the quantity of prostaglandins and leukotrienes at the site of tissue damage.

Summary

- Cell-membrane phospholipids are converted to arachidonic acid by phospholipase A_2.
- Arachidonic acid is the chemical precursor of many inflammatory mediators (eicosanoids) of which leukotrienes and prostaglandins are examples.
- Arachidonic acid is broken down into prostaglandins by the cycloxygenase enzymes.
- Prostaglandins are a family of chemicals that are also involved in pain potentiation, platelet aggregation and vascular resistance. They are absorbed by C fibres and transmitted along the axon lengths to be released within the dorsal horn.
- Substance P and CGRP are released by nociceptors into the surrounding damaged tissues which potentiates the action of the inflammatory mediators by increasing mast cell degranulation, histamine release and vasodilatation.
- The inflammatory cocktail is augmented by the release of prostaglandin I_2 and noradrenaline which is caused by the sympathetic nerve endings in the damaged tissue.
- NSAIDs and glucocorticoids (steroid drugs) inhibit the lipoxygenase and cycloxygenase enzymes and so reduce the quantity of prostaglandins and leukotrienes at the site of tissue damage (Table 1.1).

Central sensitization and Aβ fibre mediated pain

The transmission neurons within the spinal cord are subject to a barrage of impulses from peripheral nerves and from centrally descending tracts. Substance P and glutamate are released by Aδ and C fibres which act upon specific receptors on the dendrites of the transmission neurons. The receptor-neurotransmitter complex brings about depolarization of the transmission fibre which generates an

Table 1.1   Sources and actions of local hormones

Substance	Released from	Action
Hydrogen ions	Intracellular fluid	Excites nociceptors
ATP	Intracellular fluid	Acts on ATP receptors on macrophages inducing macrophage degranulation
Histamine	Macrophages, mast cells, basophils, histaminocytes (in the stomach) and histminergic neurons	Vasodilatation, increases plasma permeability. Increases gastric acid secretion. Smooth muscle contraction, with the exception of smooth muscle
Bradykinin	Cleaved from kininogens found in the tissue fluid	Activates sensory neurones, fibroblasts, endothelial cell secretion, liberates arachidonic acid
Prostaglandins	Derived from arachidonic acid by cycloxygenase	Sensitizes nociceptors to the actions of bradykinin, 5-HT and mechanical and thermal stimuli
5-IIT (serotonin)	Platelets and mast cells	Both sensitizes and activates nociceptors
Substance P	Sensory nerve endings	Induces mast cell degeneration
Leukotrienes	Derived from arachidonic acid by lipoxygenase	Sensitize nociceptors possibly by stimulating macrophages and basophils to release eicosanoids. Encourages release of substance P
Cytokines/ interleukins	Neutrophils, phagocytes	Possibly by increasing the amount of prostaglandin formation

action potential along the length of the axon. The activity of the transmission neuron is prolonged for some time after the sensory fibre has ceased firing as a result of substance P and glutamate. Also, the transmission neuron has a special excitatory amino acid receptor which is connected to an ion channel. When the transmission neuron is resting or stimulated by low-threshold sensory nerve fibres (Aβ fibres) this receptor ion channel remains inoperative, blocked by magnesium ions. The receptor ion channel can only be activated when all the ions are displaced (Mayer, Westbrook and Guthrie, 1984). This displacement of magnesium ions occurs when the transmission neuron is stimulated by an excitatory neurotransmitter such as substance P, glutamate or CGRP. The ion channel now opens and allows the influx of sodium and calcium into the neuron, producing prolonged depolarization. If another impulse arrives at the synapse before the transmission neuron slowly returns to a resting stage, another more rapid action potential is generated by the transmission neuron. Hence the transmission neuron becomes increasingly sensitive to any excitatory impulse arriving at the spinal cord. Thus the usually non-nociceptive impulses generated by Aβ fibres now produce altered sensory perception in terms of nociception.

Summary

- Modulation of the transmission neuron causes central sensitization.

- The transmission neuron has a number of receptors that are sensitive to substance P and glutamate. There is also a novel amino acid receptor which is connected to an ion channel.

- Magnesium ions block the receptor-ion channel and remains inoperative during tactile stimulation or when nociceptors are inactive.

- When magnesium is displaced, the receptor-ion channel is activated.

- When substance P, glutamate or CGRP (neurotransmitters) stimulate the transmission neuron, the displacement of magnesium can occur.

- Stimulation of the transmission neuron by neurotransmitters released from nociceptors opens the ion channel to allow influx of sodium and calcium into the neuron, producing a prolonged depolarization.

- The transmission neuron now becomes increasingly sensitive to any excitatory impulses arriving at the spinal cord, which are threfore interpreted as painful.

- The usually tactile stimulus generated by Aβ fibres now produces an altered sensory experience, felt as pain.

Now, of course we also know that pain is **individual**. Two patients who have the same condition may respond very differently: patient A is may be up and about while patient B is lying in bed, not even moving.

All of these factors are known to contribute to the individuality of the pain or the **pain threshold**, which is the amount of pain an individual is prepared to tolerate. It can vary from hour to hour or from day to day, and is influenced by a combination of the factors identified above. We also know that as health professionals we can influence this threshold in how we react to patients when they are in pain.

Here are some of the things that you probably identified (Figure 1.9):

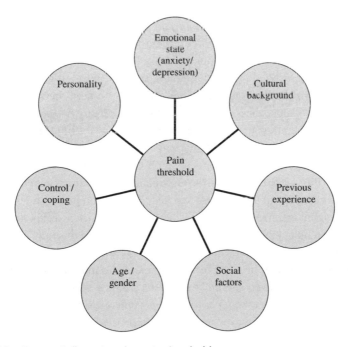

Figure 1.9　Factors influencing the pain threshold

Learning point

Consider the following statements – are they true or false?
  True / False

The attitudes of health-care staff have no effect on the patient's pain

Giving information makes the pain worse

Listening to patients' fears, previous experience and coping strategies can improve pain

Staff are in the best position to know what the patient is experiencing

All pain procedures have the same amount/level of pain

Self-medication/patient controlled analgesia make the pain worse

---

Apart from the factors that are internal to the individual, we are also influenced by those around us. For example, as carers it is important to consider how we respond to those in pain. What is the **attitude** of staff towards those in pain? Consider the place where you work and your colleagues. How do you respond to someone in pain – are you empathetic? Or do you sometimes avoid the person, maybe because you do not know what to do or say?

Many years ago Jack Hayward published *Information: A Prescription Against Pain* (1975). This work was continued by Jennifer Boore in 1978 – *Information, A Prescription for Recovery*. Both studies demonstrated that giving people information gave **control** and subsequently they were able to **cope** better. It has taken us many years to adopt these principles, but we are getting better at giving information. Think about your own clinical area – how is information given to patients/clients? Can you think of any ways that this could be improved? Is the information appropriate for older people with visual or hearing difficulties?

It is often difficult to find time to **listen** to patients. Sometimes it is easier to reach for the pharmacological approaches, and yet allowing the person to express their fears and worries is sometimes all that is needed to make them feel better. Furthermore, people tend to employ their own ways of **coping** and this may be something totally different from what you would expect, for example heat/cold or even acupuncture. Giving the person time to express their preferences may be very enlightening.

It is often said that you should be a patient to know what it is like, and this is true of pain. We cannot take a photograph of someone's pain and so we have to believe what they are telling us. As Wittgenstein (1967, p. 102) stated.

> I can only know that I am in pain – I have to accept what someone is telling me as I cannot see their pain.

How many times have you heard someone say 'Oh – they have only had their appendix removed, they shouldn't be in that much pain' or 'They should be on oral analgesics by now'. These are examples of **preconceived expectations** that are often held by nursing and medical staff, which ultimately lead to poor pain control.

Finally, there is an issue about **control** that is associated with type of analgesia. Whenever patients come into hospital, we take their medications from them and expect them to ask when they need it – of course this just makes the pain worse. Self medication systems and patient-controlled analgesia can help prevent this.

So, to summarize, all of the factors highlighted above can influence the whole pain experience. Consider a patient in your care – how many of these factors are involved in their pain experience? Both the physiological/biochemical mechanisms and the factors influencing pain form what is know as the **puzzle of pain**.

Now we have looked at the mechanisms of pain, it is useful to be able to define pain.

> Pain is what the experiencing person says it is and occurs when he/she says it does. (McCaffery, 1979 p. 95)

Do you see any problems with this definition? It has been suggested that it is a little simplistic. In addition, it requires that the individual has a command of language that we can understand. But what about those who are learning disabled, or cognitively impaired – or babies. They cannot tell us they have pain, and so traditionally they have received little attention within the literature. A more appropriate definition is that proposed by the International Association for the Study of Pain (IASP) on page 2.

Older people

Now we have discussed the physiological concepts underpinning pain processing. How does this relate to the older adult? Consider the following scenario of an elderly patient visiting her GP:

Patient	Doctor, I have pain in my leg.
GP	Oh it's to be expected at your age
Patient	But my other leg doesn't hurt and it's the same age!

This takes us back to the familiar misconceptions that are held by many people who assume that pain is to be expected as part of ageing. However, in terms of physiological changes, there is little evidence to support the fact that anything happens to the pain pathways as we get older. Although occasionally older patients may be admitted with silent myocardial infarctions or abdominal catastrophes, there is no evidence to suggest that pain pathways deteriorate with age at all. However, a number of key factors have been noted:

- Older adults tend to have reduced sensitivity to noxious stimuli, but this does not mean that when pain is present they experience it less intensely. When older adults report pain, they are likely to be afflicted with greater levels of underlying pathology than their younger counterparts who report the same level of pain (Gagliese and Melzack, 1997; Weiner and Herr, 2002).

- Older adults tend to under-report pain, because of misinterpretation of physical sensations (e.g., 'hurt' rather than 'pain'), difficulty using standard pain assessment scales, particularly in those with cognitive impairment, and false beliefs about pain and its management.

- Examples of chronic pain conditions common in adults of advanced age include osteoarthritis, postherpetic neuralgia, spinal canal stenosis, cancer, fibromyalgia, post-stroke pain and diabetic peripheral neuropathy. But is also important to remember that more than one clinical diagnosis typically contributes to chronic pain in older adults (Jones and Macfarlane, 2005) and there is also an increased likelihood of atypical pain presentations in this group, due to diminished physiological reserves and interacting co-morbidities (Helme and Gibson, 2001).

- It has been suggested that the pain in older adults tends to be constant, of moderate to severe intensity, lasting for several years, multifocal and multifactorial (Brattberg et al., 1996).

- The main problem with pain in older adults relates to impaired quality of life secondary to pain which may be expressed by depression (including increased suicide risk), anxiety, sleep disruption, appetite disturbance and weight loss, cognitive impairment, and limitations in the performance of daily activities. These added burdens are expected to improve with effective pain management (AGS Panel, 2002). Older adults with persistent pain tends to consider their health to be poorer (Reyes-Gibby, Aday and Cleeland, 2002) and use more health-care services than those without pain (Lavsky-Shulan, Wallace and Kohout, 1985).

- The prevalence rate of dementia doubles every five years from age 60 to 24% at age 70 and 30% at 85 years (Helme et al., 2003) and some suggest that the prevalence of pain appears to decrease with increased cognitive impairment. However, in patients with hip fracture, severe pain or inadequate analgesia after surgery can lead to increased confusion, slower recovery, and poorer ambulation and function (Morrison *et al.*, 2003a,b). Again there is no evidence to support the theory that pain processing changes with dementia and we should therefore treat all people the same regardless of their age or cognitive ability.

Learning Point

Can you write down a situation from your practice whereby you perceived an older person with/without cognitive impairment to be in pain?

- How was this situation handled by the staff?
- How did you know this person was in pain?
- What have you learned from this?
- How will you deal with the situation differently in the future based upon your new knowledge?

Many of us know when someone is experiencing pain, and we need to be confident in our perception and deal with it. Of course we talk about being the patient's advocate, and recognizing pain and doing something about it is fundamental to the principals of advocacy:

- Recognizing pain-provoking situations.
- Pre-empting pain.
- Fostering a multidisciplinary approach to pain management.

Conclusion

Our understanding of the physiology of pain remains rudimentary, particularly in scientific terms. The relationship between the pain pathways and the higher centres within the brain remains uncertain. The concept of individuality or threshold also complicates the picture. Think of the disproportionate pain caused by something minor such as a paper cut – and yet we often see major injuries that do not appear to produce much pain. The physiology of pain is important, but only goes some way to explain the phenomenon. Scientists, clinicians and researchers are in agreement that further work needs to be done.

Understanding the physiology of pain is essential if practitioners are going to be in a position to prescribe appropriate analgesics or other forms of treatment.

Pain is a common symptom of disease, and the one problem that drives individuals to seek help.

The population is getting older, and we are likely to see increasing numbers of older adults who are experiencing pain. It is essential therefore, that healthcare professionals are aware of the basic principals of physiology and the pain pathways to enable them to understand and deal with the problems. The gate control theory remains our primary theory of pain and stands the test of time, so familiarity with this theory will help us to understand pain and apply appropriate management strategies.

*All figures taken from Drago (2005) and adapted by Matthew Schofield.

References

AGS Panel on Persistent Pain in Older Persons (2002) The management of persistent pain in older persons. *Journal of the American Geriatric Society*, **6**(Suppl), S205–24.

Brain, S.D. and Williams, T.J. (1985) Inflammatory oedema induced by synergism between calcitonin gene related peptide and mediators of increased vascular permeability. *British Journal of Pharmacology*, **86**, 855–60.

Brattberg, G., Parker, M.G. and Thorslund, M. (1996) The prevalence of pain among the oldest old in Sweden. *Pain*, **67**, 29–34.

Cesare, P. and McNaughton, P. (1997) Peripheral pain mechanisms. *Current Opinion in Neurology*, **7**, 493–9.

Davis, P. (1993) Opening up the gate control theory. *Nursing Standard* **7**, 25–7.

Davis, B.D. (2000) *Caring for People in Pain*. Routledge, London.

Dickenson, A. (2002) Gate control theory of pain stands the test of time. *British Journal of Anaesthesia* Editorial I. 88.6 755–7.

Fields, H.L. and Basbaum A.L. (1994) Central nervous system mechanisms of pain modulation, in *Textbook of Pain* (eds P. Wall and R. Melzack), Churchill Livingstone, Edinburgh.

Gagliese, L. and Melzack, R. (1997) Chronic pain in elderly people. *Pain*, **70**, 3–14.

Helme, R.D. and Katz, B. (2003) Chronic pain in the elderly, in *Clinical Pain Manaagment: Chronic Pain* (ed. A. Rice *et al.*), Arnold, London.

Jones, G.T. and Macfarlane, G.J. (2005) Epidemiology of pain in older persons, in *Pain in Older Persons. Progress in Pain Research and Management*, vol. 35, (eds S.J. Gibson and D.K. Weiner), pp. 3–23. IASP Press, Seattle.

Lavsky-Shulan, M., Wallace, R.B. and Kohout, F.J. (1985) Prevalence and functional correlates of low back pain in the elderly: the Iowa 65+ rural health study. *Journal of the American Geriatric Society*, **33**, 23–8.

McCaffery, M. (1979) *Nursing Management for the Patient with Pain*, J.B. Lippincott, Co., New York.

Mayer, M.L., Westbrook, G. and Guthrie, P.B. (1984) Voltage-dependent block by magnesium of NMDA responses to spinal cord neurons. *Nature*, **309**, 261–3.

Melzack, R. and Wall, P. (1965) Pain mechanisms: a new theory. *Science*, **150**, 971–9.

Melzack, R. and Wall, P. (1996) *The Challenge of Pain*, 2nd edn. Penguin, London.

Merskey, H. (ed.) (1986) Classification of chronic pain: descriptions of chronic pain syndromes and definitions of pain terms. *Pain Supplement*, **3**, S1–255.

Merskey, H. and Bogduk, N. (1992) *Taxonomy of Pain Terms and Definitions*, IASP Press, Seattle.

Morrison, R.S., Magaziner, J. and Gilbert, M. *et al.* (2003a) Relationship between pain and opioid analgesics on the development of delirium following hip fracture. *Journal of Gerontology*, **58**, 76–81.

Morrison, R.S., Magaziner, J. and McLaughlin, M.A. *et al.* (2003b) The impact of post-operative pain on outcomes following hip fracture. *Pain*, **103**, 303–11.

Mountcastle, V.B (1980) *Medical Physiology*, Mosby, St Louis.

Rang, H.P., Dale, M.M., and Ritter, J.M. (1999) *Pharmacology*, 4th edition, Churchill Livingstone, Edinburgh.

Reyes-Gibby, C.C., Aday, L. and Cleeland, C. (2002) Impact of pain on self-rated health in the community-dwelling older adults. *Pain*, **95**, 75 82.

Wall P.D. and Melzack R. (ed.) (1999) *Textbook of Pain*, 4th edn. Churchill Livingstone, Edinburgh.

Weiner, D.K. and Herr, K (2002) Comprehensive interdisciplinary assessment and treatment planning: an integrated overview, in *Persistent Pain in Older Adults: An Interdisciplinary Guide for Treatment* (eds D.K. Weiner, K. Herr and T.E. Rudy), pp. 18–57. Springer, New York.

Wells, J.C.D. and Woolf, C.J. (ed.) (1991) Pain mechanisms and management. *British Medical Bulletin*, **47**, 3.

Willer, J.C. (1979) Comparative study of perceived pain and nociceptive influx in man. *Pain*, **3**, 69–80.

Wittgenstein, L. (1967) *The Philosophical Investigations*. Anchor Books, New York.

Woolf, C.J. (1989) Recent advances in the pathophysiology of acute pain. *British Journal of Anaesthesia*, **63**, 139–46.

Woolf, C.J. (1991) Generations of acute pain: central mechanisms. *British Medical Bulletin*, **47**, 523–33.

Relating socio-economic issues to older people and pain: independence, dignity and choice

2

Mary Cooke

Introduction

This chapter aims to look at how older people's personal expectations influence their socio-economic situation, and how this affects their adaptation to their personal situation. The review includes socio-economic issues in understanding the debilitating effects of older age and pain, and the perception of pain in complex conditions. The literature draws upon information about the older population in Britain, with reflections on other cultures. The key issues for older people in the 21st century are examined, reflecting policies linked to multicultural attitudes to old age and evaluating the effectiveness of resources on attitudes to pain prevention as part of managing complex long-term conditions. Issues and policies associated with age, income and education are reviewed, as well as the physical and mental health management of older people by diet, medication and activity. Before this, we look at aspects of economics that link to health, and issues related to health policy that directly influence older people's experiences.

The chapter is made up of three main sections. In the first section we look at the expectation of economic independence in older age, and compare this with economic dependence based on the importance of pain control or alleviation as a benchmark. In the next section, in association with understanding the role of a person's economic status and control over their health, we examine the issue of dignity in old age and how assumptions are made on behalf of the older population, society and individuals. Finally, we look at how economic choices are set for older people, what these choices are based on, and whether opportunities to alter health status in old age can be selected.

Economics, health, age and independence

That health decreases with age (normally) is a fundamental fact of biology (Buckley *et al.*, 2004). Because age is frequently correlated with income, education and other variables, it is essential to control for age through age-adjustment, or analysis of age-specific data (Contoyannis and Jones, 2004).

Gender differential in life expectancy

Interactions between age and other variables such as income and education become important; in particular, the correlation between health and income varies greatly over the life cycle, and not monotonically. At the close of the 20th century, the life expectancy of women exceeded that of men in every country. This is attributable to biological differences, but interactions between these differences and the physical and social environment vary. In low-income countries ($1000 gross domestic product [GDP] per capita or less) the female–male difference in life expectancy is only about 4%. For countries with GDP per capita around $3000 it is 8%, and at around $9000 it averages 11%. However, the differential does not follow this path continuously. In the 30 highest income countries (GDP per capita averaging $21,000) the gender differential in life expectancy is only 8%.

Over the past 30 years the differential in higher-income countries has tended to fall, reversing the previous long-term trend towards a higher ratio in the course of economic development. In the United States, for example, the downward trend occurred at the same time that the female–male education ratio was rising (ONS, 2006; Fuchs, 2004). Over age 65 the sex ratio has for a long time been 49% male 51% female, but this percentage is shifting to indicate that more men live longer. The needs of the elderly population will alter in response to this. Pensions and benefits are already adjusted to support people living longer on average by 10 years than they did 20 years ago. Currently decisions are being made to raise the age of retirement for the fit elderly, so that pensions and welfare benefits are given to those who are unable to support themselves in older age, while others can contribute more towards their retirement for when they choose to cease work. The economic benefits to older people of working longer are not yet quantified.

Health economics

Health economics is a way of expressing a personal and social value for health and health services. The unique British National Health Service (NHS) provides health care free at the point of delivery for people who need it. For people over 60 years, this also means free prescriptions, eye tests and other benefits.

People who need health care decide with their GP when and where this will happen.

The point at which the cost of care becomes important is when people are willing and able to pay for treatment. In the UK people may choose either to pay for care, or have NHS care. Most interventions and treatments have an outcomes-related benefit. This means that the cost related to effectiveness or benefit is calculated on various characteristics of patients and the treatment, to suggest whether an intervention is likely to be effective, beneficial or too costly. In the UK there are standardized reference costs of interventions linked to people aged under and over 70 years, giving the cost of a bed used per day, an expected length of stay per treatment, and the intervention. Currently, nine strategic (regional) health authorities hold the budget for treatments in the NHS. Several systems help make the decision along with the patient about what treatment is available, whether the budget will pay for the intervention, and what is likely to be a good outcome for the patient and for society generally. Sometimes people may not get the treatment they need when they need it because the resources have been spent (**opportunity costs**). This is called **rationing, resource allocation** or **budget management**. Balancing available resources (staff, technology, equipment and money as income from various sources) with the needs of people in a local population is the basis of economic science. Individuals' values for health and local health services are the criteria for decisions about health spending and health policies that control health-care delivery.

Cultural issues in older age

The rise in the number of people over 60 years old in most western societies in recent years has important implications for western cultures and their social construct. Life expectancy is 7 years less for black Americans than for white Americans, and possibly greater for Hispanics than for white Americans, but the reasons for this are not understood (Fuchs, 2004). The health services of many countries, including Australia, the Balkan states, Canada, Finland, Greece, Israel, Italy, Japan, Poland, Spain, Sweden,Taiwan, Turkey, the UK and the USA, are beginning to recognize the impact of the needs of older people when considering cultural aspects of illness prevention by nutrition, controlling pain and symptoms of long-term illness and disease by 'safe' analgesia, and prevention of pain through symptom recognition. Fuchs (2004) suggests that interactions between genes and socio-economic variables exist. For example social scientists often cite stress as a major cause of bad health, but sceptics found that effects of apparently the same stressors vary across individuals. Inherited genetic factors associated with varying levels of depression are inherent in each individual to their old age. These factors cross all race and ethnic demographic features and correlate with how an individual adapts to change which then affects related health issues. Most people's cost of care rises dramatically in the last six months of life Sheshamani and Gray,

2004), mainly because of heroic treatments and increased hospital episodes of care. Older people's genetic and ethnic differences become more pronounced for pain control, but in the UK analgesia is not selected according to race, or cost.

Long-term, complex chronic illness is the norm for many people over 50 in the UK and other countries. The ease of international travel means that older people from many cultures visit or live in the UK, and they may have different ways of thinking about older age. In countries such as Ukraine, for example, average life expectancy is 67 years, whereas in the UK it is 84 years (ONS, 2006). There are cultural differences too: in Japan and other Asian countries older people are venerated and cared for in their family home until death. In Asian cultures, 'old' may mean over 45 years of age. These key culture-specific issues provide different perspectives for many British older people, and particularly those who have moved from other cultures to live here. Costs for families with ill older members differ in accordance with cultural influences.

Analysis of the causes of inequalities in health has shown that variation in the utilization of medical care cannot fully explain observed health differences (Auster, Levenson and Sarachek, 1969; Evans, Barer and Marmor, 1994). Epidemiologists, sociologists and economists have indicated that lifestyle contributes to these inequalities. It is personal lifestyle that causes the greatest variation, beyond a low level of food, hygiene and basic health-care provision. McGinnis and Foege (1993) estimated that the three leading external (non-degenerative or directly genetically determined) causes of mortality in the USA in 1990 were tobacco, diet and activity, and alcohol consumption. These lifestyle variables explained around 38% of premature mortality, and the researchers noted that a dramatically reduced quality of life is associated with many of the diseases related to these behaviours (Contoyannis and Jones, 2004).

The impact of disability arising from poor pain control is the same in the UK as it is internationally. Epidemiological outcomes of interventions and planning for illness prevention in care of the elderly and their personal infirmities are based on the individuals' inherited poverty or wealth, their nutritional habits, their lifetime opportunities taken through education, their manner of resource use, and their resulting health status. This is sometimes called the **social capital** of a community, meaning its wealth of health and ability to maintain independence.

Summary

- The UK is a multicultural society.
- Pain control is just as poor in the UK as in other countries.
- People's health in old age is dependent upon their intrinsic health status at birth, their education, and their lifestyle during youth and mid-life.

Resources linked with being older and in pain

While they are still young and active, few people expect or plan for the experiences of chronic pain, illness and complex diseases of old age, or for the personal costs of support required. This means that few resources are forthcoming from individuals themselves, except learned coping strategies for pain or adaptation. The effect of chronic pain on each individual's daily life will cause them to adjust their activity by adapting to the changing problems of mobility, diet, activity and an individual expectation of successful adoption of personal coping strategies tested through life experience. Relative fitness and frailty can be defined by accumulation of physical deficits until the person is unable to improve health by medical or other treatment. Mitnitski *et al.* (2005) state that 'there are maximal values of deficit accumulation beyond which survival is unlikely'. Several studies recognize that health-care staff's attitudes and methods of communication in the community setting are associated with recognizing individual's needs arising from complex conditions, and where personal coping and management strategies are important (Schofield *et al.*, 2005, p. 20).

Older people cite methods of coping with pain that include spending time with friends and family, reading and watching television, rest, and favourite old folk remedies. Some of these remedies require financial resources such as funds for transport or for treatments that are not part of NHS care.

Other studies show that pain in older age influences mental health status (Muira *et al.*, 2004; Muira, Ari and Yamasaki, 2005), and attitude towards food and nutrition or even access to health care (Litaker and Love, 2005). Most people over 60 in the UK will have lived through the Second World War and its aftermath, when they experienced rationing of food and goods. The wartime diet was high in fibre and vegetables, but after rationing ended foods that were low in fibre and high in fat and sugar became part of the diet again. The rise in cancer of the colon in people over 50 years, which is affected by diet, may be the cost to society of this change.

For most older people, medication for pain is taken as a last resort, mainly because of the attitude of health-care staff towards 'strong' medication, and also because of the side effects of continuous analgesic use (Schofield *et al.*, 2005, p. 13) The variety of the coping mechanisms listed above indicates that they achieve something other than reduction of pain by the older person, based to an extent on their culture, level of independence, maintenance of personal dignity and choices available in the use of resources (Litaker and Love, 2005). These resources are considered to be personal (coping methods learned through life experiences), financial (income), and interdependent decision-making with regard to access and choice of methods of pain reduction. Older people use a hierarchy of symptom control and contact with health or social care services (Schofield *et al.*, 2005, p. 97; Gustafsson, Ekblad and Sidenvall, 2005) with an intention of avoiding expenditure of personal financial resources. It is noticed that older people do not want to take on long-term costs of long-term pain management.

It is inevitable that rates of morbidity and mortality increase with age, reflecting the ongoing deterioration of health. Buckley *et al.* (2004) modelled the influences of socio-economic factors on the state of health of older Canadians. The Canadian system offers universal access to a publicly funded health-care system that covers 'essential services', which (in the late 1990s) meant about 70% of all health expenditure on services. The income–health connection has been reviewed in depth by, for example, Smith (1999); Evans (2002); Deaton (2002, 2003). One conclusion of this literature is that

> the determinants of health indicate that at least among citizens of wealthy societies, any relationship between individual income level and health status has to arise from the effects of the social context within which people at different levels find themselves. Income inequality, like air pollution, is itself a health hazard. However, it is not certain that income inequality itself is a major determinant of population health . . . . [I]t is low incomes that are important, not inequality and there is no evidence that making the rich richer . . . is hazardous to the health of the poor. (Buckley *et al.*, 2004, p. 3).

Lifetime income affects both men and women. Higher income means greater command over resources, including greater access to adequate nutrition. It could also affect access to health care; even in a universal system some elements of care (e.g. prescription drugs, access to health-care professionals such as physiotherapists) or the private costs of accessing the systems (such as transport costs) are not covered. The system may be too 'downstream' – concerned with health-related behaviour and health-care delivery and drugs – when the underlying 'causes of causes' of diseases and death are more 'upstream' in the social and economic structure of society. The treatments for complex conditions and pain control lie within this layered structure (Deaton, 2002, p. 14).

Summary

- Chronic pain from illness and complex conditions in older age is often untreated.
- Older people from all cultures do not always access health services to treat pain, sometimes because of staff attitudes to medication.
- Life experiences, culture-specific remedies and maintenance of independence promote an adaptation to pain in older people.
- Income while working is a factor influencing men's and women's health in older age.

Policy in health services, economics and older people

The National Service Framework (NSF) for Older People was published by the Labour Government in 2001 (DH, 2001) as one of a series of frameworks for modernizing health services with a focus on managing people's health needs in a community setting.

This NSF requires the setting up and maintenance of a network of services for older people to be purchased and managed from primary care trusts (PCTs), with links for social services to deliver social care when appropriate. A PCT in a region or area takes the lead on managing services for the elderly. Other related non-disease-specific NSFs have been set up, such as the NSF for Long Term Conditions (DH, 2005). Adult-focused NSFs have also been issued for specific conditions or diagnoses such as cancer, heart disease, diabetes and asthma. A successful NSF is seen as being interactive between patients, health-care staff and social services, using available resources to benefit local populations and interlinking various health-enhancing services as required by local groups representative of elderly people.

The social context of shared benefits in health is shown in a Danish study (Gyrd-Hansen, 2004). In this study equity was traded off for greater health gains, and related to whether the questions in the survey were framed to elicit a social or an individual choice. If social decision-making is the issue, health gains which involve relieving patients of extreme problems are found to be valued more highly than relief of minor ailments. This is a defined value system for making decisions affecting personal health and comfort.

The practical physical and psychosocial limitations of pain confronting older people are dealt with by strategies for maintaining independence and control, and adaptation to life with chronic pain (Sofaer et al., 2005). Navigating systems of access to health care is a mystery to most older people, although one third of them suffer chronic pain and live in fear of losing their independence. Many participants in Sofaer's study used adaptation, acceptance or non-acceptance of their condition, but by pacing themselves, helping others, prayer, and using a 'public face' they were able to overcome the pain (Sofaer et al., 2005). Such strategies are anticipated to be cost free for the older people using them and for the state, but this attitude determines the value older people have for their independence.

Policies for GPs and community drug prescribers have recently been associated with reducing the costs of prescription drugs. Insufficient pain management in the community and in acute settings is a public health concern, and adequate relief depends upon a variety of treatment options including the appropriate use of controlled substances for moderate or severe pain. In the UK the use of opioids in pain management is regulated by local health authorities, and is the concern of GPs and specialist nurses who alter dose and rate in the individual's home or hospice according to need. Research in the USA (Gilson, Maurer and Joranson, 2005; Guglielmo, 2006) identifies concerns about older people having state-controlled substances in their homes, and being vulnerable to theft or diversion and abuse of drugs by family or health-care staff. In the UK, current policies support the reduction in length of hospital stay, and rehabilitation and treatment are focused on the home setting. Future policies will concern pain management and strategies to intended reduce crime in the community.

Diet and health in older age, related to economics

Disease-related diet and information (for example sugar-free foods for diabetics, fresh fruit and vegetables for raising energy and reducing depression, protein and vitamin-rich foods for wound healing) may inform but not influence an individual's compliance with advice. Older people in the UK have experienced many countervailing arguments around food and food products, so confusion in popular and cultural notions of the 'right' food to eat is likely. Food interests may not be related to health interests, and information relating to pain reduction through promoting mental health may be inaccessible. Gustafsson, Ekblad and Sidenvall (2005) show that within a culture members often eat foods specific to that culture (Douglas, 1966) because the meaning of eating healthily for older people may not always be to eat a variety of foods including fresh meat and vegetables. For others, this is seen as 'proper food' (Dickinson, 1999). Hirani and Primatesta's study (2005) shows significantly that older people (over 65) living in institutions and at home risk poor bone and muscle health and increased risk of fractures because of low vitamin D levels. Deficiency is more likely to be found in women than in men, is more likely in the autumn and winter, and is associated with long limiting illness, manual social class and poor general health. Vitamin D is an indicator of healthy exposure to daylight and sunlight coupled with a diet containing fish and fortified dairy and cereal products.

Food choice is influenced by socio-economic factors, level of education and whether an individual lives independently or in an institution. Allen's study (2005) indicates that based on personal resources, even the presence of an elderly individual's own teeth has a significant effect on dental treatment, because of cost, and on diet. Easily chewed food items with a low fibre and high fat content may increase their risk of cardiovascular disease and bowel cancer. Current dietary choices using similar content are based on cost rather than perceived quality (Gustafsson and Sidenvall, 2002). This provides health and social care professionals with important information about individual dietary influences on the health of the local population.

The differences in adjustment made by women in old age who will have experienced many life changes, and possibly hardship, are explored (Traynor, 2005). She found that depression, maintaining intimacy through friends and managing change are the key influences on women's perceptions of health and pain management. Distress related to poverty, and the need for social and emotional support, become important for women in older life, who may be widowed or whose family may no longer be close enough to provide a financial or social cushion. Family ties become important when government policy changes benefits assessments, pension rights, investments, and taxable allowances for older people's incomes. Information about pensions, welfare and benefits income, or support through voluntary and public services is not universally available, and an older person who is isolated will be disadvantaged, possibly in debt, and with a reduced standard of living.

The independence of older people is often associated with the availability and use of transport. Having no personal transport, and thus lacking access to local shops and therefore to fresh produce, is associated with low income and poor education. Older drivers will become more prevalent because of the large post-war social cohort, and it is predicted that future older drivers will drive greater distances and take more trips (OECD, 2001). Statistically older people are safer drivers, but the presence of more older drivers will increase the morbidity and mortality of people involved in road traffic accidents (Hakamies-Blomqvist, Wiklund and Henriksson, 2005).

Dignity associated with older age is usually linked to assessment of need for services and predictions of ageing populations. Assessment of frailty may or may not be helpful (Duke, 2006). To avoid allocating a person to a category from which they cannot escape may require several sequential assessments – costly, time-consuming and inconvenient – to reduce the risk that expediency might override fairness.

The safety of older people living at home is normally ignored. In the USA unintentional injuries are the ninth leading cause of death in people aged 65 and older, and for every death there are 650 non-fatal injuries (Cresci, 2005). Two studies indicate that costs of care increase through the last 15 years before death. The association between age and health expenditure may well be an artefact of a stronger relationship between proximity to death and health expenditure, as mentioned above (Sheshamani and Gray, 2004; Lagergren, 2005). Lagergren also makes the point that guidance of the provision of health services for older people requires better data to make predictions associated with need. Cost reduction in older age is linked to policy measures directed at improving the health of elderly people by promoting conditions of increased physical and mental activity and better outcomes for medical interventions (Lagergren, 2005).

Choice in how to maintain a reasonable income while older and retired from mainstream work is a current debate in many countries, relating to pensions, ability to work and health. In Ukraine older people, if they live beyond the average of 67 years, will take up laborious jobs on the streets to make ends meet. Because Ukrainian health policies are weak, people turn to folk medicine and Eastern medications to treat illnesses, or emigrate to obtain western health care (Lipsitz, 2005). Older poor rural Chinese who have lived through the transition from Communism to private health insurance mostly have to pay directly for health care, which means that only 6.1% of them access services (Wang *et al.*, 2005).

Poverty in old age is related to the person's ability to adapt to their reduction in income, or choose to move. Health status is associated with physical and mental health, mobility, and accrued investment during working life. Long-term benefits and state pensions form a baseline income but reduce mental health further, with a risk of early entry to the care-home setting (Crist, 2005; Okoro *et al.*, 2005; Polansky and Smoyak, 2005; Janlov, Hallberg and Petersson, 2006). The alternative is to accommodate health needs to health expectations. Policies assume that older people will be independent as long as possible (Crist, 2005), which reduces costs of health care Sheshamani and Gray (2004). Personal dignity is lost when older people can no longer choose their destiny because of personal resources, government policy, or local application of social rules that are applied to regulate the cost of illness to society (Byford, Torgerson and Raftery, 2000).

Summary

- Reducing symptoms causing pain in older people is based on individual understanding and experiences of what they will 'lose' by going to the doctor, (opportunity costs of using health services) rather than what they will gain. Health policies in other parts of the world increase health inequalities of immigrants to the UK.

- Older people have learned habits of using few resources that are difficult to change.

- Some cultures consider 'old' to be around 50 years, others venerate older people aged 80 or more. These cultural differences are noticed more when people go without health care because they think it costs money.

- Past events such as wars affect people's attitudes to what they can or should eat, shape opinions on the cost of things and affect the ability to access fresh produce.

Independence

People who are older and living independently have a healthier and longer life if they are not depressed (Cully *et al.*, 2005). Physical ill-health, as well as any indication of loss of mental health, contributes to a gradual rise in dependence and loss of ability to make decisions independent of family and others upon whom the older person may depend. Physical health can be assessed in several ways: here we use temperature, fitness, safety, diet, depression and understanding of diagnosis as markers for independence.

Many older people have to decide whether to leave their family home and move to live in a care home, or with younger family members. Van Houtven and Norton identified factors that reduced the need for or introduction of home health care, and delayed nursing home entry significantly.

Depression is an underlying condition for many older adults, and predicts their ability to adapt to changes in health status (Cully *et al.*, 2005) and rehabilitation after a stroke or other episodes of illness. There are few studies that clarify the effect of depression on the in-patient rehabilitation process. Once depression is apparent the functional deficits associated with its occurrence persist, even after remission of the depressive episode. If two populations of in-patients with and without stroke are compared, their clinically meaningful symptoms of depression are similar. This is because there are underlying complications of managing a chronic illness or condition. Nahcivan and Demirezen (2005) have shown that more than 50% of the population of older adults living on low incomes in a rural community setting in Turkey suffer symptoms of depression. This half of the population is more likely to be women or widows, to lack health insurance and to live alone. The psycho-social aspect of pain associated with being older is partly linked with income and social standing, and closely linked with coping and resources. Older people in the UK from various cultures often assume they have to pay for services that are actually free, and this means they do not receive some aspects of care.

Informal care given by family members complements professional care or substitutes for it, but this care is not conducive to the long-term interests of the individual family member who becomes the chief carer. Muira, Ari and Yamasaki (2005) show the burden of caring on spouses and the co-morbidity linked with reduction in quality of life because of mental capacity and verbal communication. The relationship between depression and anxiety among long-term caregivers and their feelings of burden are succinctly linked here. Previous work indicated that social activity added value to quality of relationship. This requires an element of resource use, and consequent funds to accommodate this activity (Muira *et al.*, 2004). The influence of depression when linked to independent living is applied to core body temperature and reflects the use of resources. Gomolin *et al.* (2005) used this phenomenon in a study that showed older people in a nursing home setting were colder than those living independently in the community. In fact older people were colder in all settings: nursing home, office and community than younger people in the same environment. This means that older people have a lower average core body temperature, which is not often recognised when recording baseline observations.

Independence in older age assumes that a person is living in the community in their own home setting, either alone or with at least one other person. Further, it means that resources defined as financial (pension, benefits, interest on savings and investments) and personal (health, education and knowledge about their condition, ability to decide about or pay for treatments) have been accrued by the person during their life, and are now being used to their benefit in older age.

The study by Hirani and Primatesta (2005) shows in a large cross-sectional sample (n = 1766) that vitamin D is an indicator of older people's ability to access or afford fish and fortified dairy or cereal products, or even appreciate the benefit of vegetables and fruit in the diet. Many older people are physically unable to prepare vegetables, or find cooking costly. Older people's inability to provide themselves with an adequate diet will eventually affect their independence.

Cresci (2005) describes the use of a Cochrane systematic review to underpin assessment of elderly home safety. The home care nurse, as a key member of the team, raises awareness of extrinsic and intrinsic factors that may lead to injury in the home, and suggest strategies for injury prevention. Home safety resources (local, state and internet) and the personal injury plan are part of an education process. The lack of independence is outlined by the process of accumulated health-related problems (deficits) defined by Mitnitski *et al.* (2005), as mentioned earlier. Here the team use an index of frailty in older adults and mortality in population-based and clinical/institutional-based samples to identify a hazard rate for mortality from a level of accumulated ill health.

Dignity

Even in the UK, health care is bound by finances and a managed market. This means that for the providers in the health-care system – GPs and secondary or acute health care organizations – patients can be seen as income, or at least income generating. Economic management of health care and services is part of the managed market in health. Success depends on the understanding of raising resource income and reducing expenditures, to ensure income is greater than expenditure. Investment in health enhancing features can reduce resource use in the long term. So health promoting behaviours practiced by patients are usually encouraged. A healthy older person (a consumer) has a capitation fee, and a fee for service, which raises each GP's income, whereas an ill 'patient' is costly. A study by Iversen identified the active recruitment of patients by GPs if they experienced a reduction in income. This perception of the patient as income has not been explicitly expressed previously (Iversen, 2004).

In contrast, patients can decide to use private health care. The current state of the NHS, characterized by long waits and generally poor quality, has driven many to spend savings accrued for precautionary reasons. Guariglia and Rossi (2004) found a correlation between insurance coverage and saving in the UK, suggesting that private medical insurance does not generally crowd out private saving, yet preserves the dignity of having health care when and where it is important to the individual.

The study by Janlov *et al.* (2006) indicates the loss of dignity and 'walking a fine line' while balancing the feelings of guilt and need for comfort against resources when deciding on accepting 'a necessary evil' by incorporating the home help into daily life to gain a sense of continuity. The assessment of personal wealth under these circumstances has the effect of reducing control over resources, because giving information away in relation to wealth provides others – even if they are anonymous public agencies – with a means by which an individual is measured, and their capacity associated with their ability to pay rather than their willingness to pay for services.

Barnes and Bennet (1998) and Roberts (2001, 2002) found that older people in later life who are increasingly frail because of disease and co-morbidity are vulnerable when exercising their right to participate in and influence decisions relating to their own health and social care. Older people experienced countervailing pressures by health staff either through assessments of needs before admission to an institution, or assessment of ability before discharge. This assessment is entirely professional-led, taking little account of the patient- or person-centred approach favoured by current policies.

There is little attempt to understand the functioning of the NHS as an institution in a study by Campbell *et al.* (2005) describing predictors of clinical outcomes from a European collaborative group, measuring physical function, cognition, age, gender and living arrangement as a factors associated with outcome. There was little recognition that the NHS and social care system often prevents the older person from leaving the institution within the 90 day 'deadline' for institutionalization (Gray and Martin, 2005).

Summary

- Economics balances expenses and costs with income, and has little to do with the dignity of the individual seen by some as an enhancement to fees or income.
- Accepting help at home by older people is seen as becoming less independent and a burden on family.
- Assessment of needs associated with cost is a process centred on health professionals and not on the person about whom decisions will be made.

Choice

Understanding generations can be enhanced by avoiding defining them rigidly as chronological cohorts, but rather linking generational experiences with a historically informed political economy. The 'War generation' recognizes itself and therefore has a common identity, with values, attitudes and sense of national solidarity and mutual obligation arising from those experiences. However, the generation is divided by divergent economic interests in property, insurance protection and pension rights, based on historical experiences of life course by experienced groups. Some would identify the choices they had in developing financial opportunities, others deny they had a choice of life experience (Vincent, 2005). Inevitably, selecting financial gain early in life indicated better health outcomes and greater independence in older age (Van Hootven and Norton, 2004).

The construction of the National Insurance system in the UK is intended for the benefit of all, yet clearly older people are expected to use a greater proportion of their financial resources in accessing and using the NHS, as well as subsidizing it by the use of other methods of health maintenance for pain and symptom control or reduction (Schofield *et al.*, 2005, p. 69) This raises the question whether older people choose to use the health service, or choose to put off accepting help with pain relief as long as possible. The reduction in pain can be either physical (Sofaer *et al.*, 2005); Cully *et al.*, 2005) or mental, as described by Muira, Ari and Yamasaki (2005). A study by Wang *et al.* (2005) shows that across most populations the poorer populations subsidize the rich/sick in utilization of health services, which counters the findings of Buckley *et al.* (2004). This idea is upheld by Le Grand (1991, 2003) who indicates that health policy intended to help the poor and sick cannot acknowledge the needs of that population without the rich and sick taking advantage of the health provision to the detriment of those needy poor.

Outpatient and in-patient services use by a poor rural community are modelled by Wang *et al.* (2005) based on income and health status. These authors made an assumption that if individuals consume more non-medical goods then they have capacity to pay for more health care, and this reflects people's ability to pay. The health status of any given population has been shown to have a positive relationship with the standard of education of that population, although this does not take account of the risk-taking behaviour of members of that population.

Lipsitz (2005) writes of a Ukrainian population where 15% are aged over 65 years, despite the average length of life being only 67 years. The ratio of older women to men is 2:1, and the presence of elderly women is so ubiquitous that they even have a special word (*babushka*) to describe them. As in most other cultures, the incidence of poverty increases with age and 49% of households with two or more elderly people are considered to be poor, because the average pension is 40%

below the poverty line, based on an annual household consumption of $24 per month. This is why the most vulnerable segment of the population seemingly provides much of the hard labour in Ukrainian cities. During the Soviet era health care was free as a public service, although standards were and are considered lower than in western health care. Central and eastern European countries collectively report reduction in real income and widening disparities, because of stress and stress-related behaviour (e.g. consumption of alcohol and tobacco) lax regulation of environmental and occupational risks, and breakdown in basic health services.

Preventive care is rare in the Ukraine, because of the proportion of resources allocated to community and ambulatory care. The high cost of drugs prevents older people from affording lipid-lowering medications, modern antihypertensive medication, calcium, vitamin D or even aspirin. The system is able to provide only rudimentary acute care, despite spending two thirds of health funds on secondary services which are highly specialized but poorly equipped, with minimal nursing care and little heating. Because of the high prevalence of drug abuse in the population (a result of social and psychological pressures) there is limited access to modern psychiatric care. Depression, anxiety and psychoses therefore often remain untreated in frail elderly patients unable to travel far for treatment. Opiate analgesics are strictly regulated in the Ukraine, and are generally unavailable except to patients with end-stage cancer. Most of the elderly population treat themselves with herbs, folk medicine and devices they can make themselves or purchase cheaply in local pharmacies, according to long-standing cultural practices and beliefs based on specific treatment or behaviour for every symptom. Many families travel and migrate with their elderly relatives to countries with better-developed health services such as the UK of Germany. The description of conditions in the Ukraine is given here to indicate the similarities of belief by older people in health care and lack of preventive health care that exists between the UK and the Ukraine.

The continuing increase in the use of complementary medicines in many western countries indicates that people of all ages are making positive choices between allopathic and complementary health approaches. NHS prescriptions are free for people over 60 in the UK, so the cost of complementary therapies may not be prohibitive when culture-specific remedies are required. A specific study of older people's use of complementary medications in the USA indicated a growth in use similar to that in the UK (25% over the last 20 years). The study showed that out-of-pocket expenditure on complementary therapies by older people was more than that spent on hospitalization (Shreffler-Grant et al., 2005).

The use of health services is greater by older people in the population than by others, except that the proportion of people who are educated and more wealthy access health care more frequently. This selective inverse use of services influences the GDP per capita in the UK. Older people do not always choose to use health services; their attitude towards pain and seeking help appears to be laissez-faire. A decision not to access services is not always based on ability or willingness to pay for medication; rather, a choice to go without is associated with an ability to make that choice, or else the system in the UK is so complex that navigating it is too difficult. In countries where resources to pay for health care and pain relief are low, older people counteract their lack of pain relief by work. In the UK, a comprehensive approach to meeting the health-care needs of the older population comes from understanding the older person's perception of pain.

Summary

- Older people are expected to use the health services more than other sectors of the population.

- Health professionals often implicitly place restrictions on older people's choice of interventions for treatments. The older people tend to pay for complementary therapies to treat pain.

- People from poorer countries migrate to welfare-based health economies to gain better health care and pain relief if they can.

- Health risk-taking at a younger age reflects an attitude to health in older age, but is linked to the ability to pay for services.

Conclusion

The spectrum of social capital and health among older people in the UK ranges from personal investment in health by reducing their acknowledgement of pain or enhancing life through lifestyle, to loss of independence and lack of choice about health interventions, and to depression. This continuum indicates that dignity is an important factor. Social capital may function on several levels, through individual behaviours (such as community participation) individual norms (trust in the community and perceptions of community reciprocity), through the neighbourhood environment, and is defined at the macro level by historical, social, political and economic features. Changes in abilities to partici-pate mean that the older person or group comes to depend upon social capital at each of these points (Canniscio *et al.*, 2003 Pollack and von dem Knesebeck, 2004). The recognition that older people will either be living at home, or in a supported care environment, means that the quality of life in either setting will become more important. Personal expectations of each older person resonate with their health status and ability to communicate needs and choices. Symptoms and dependency will reduce quality of life, even though 'cure' is impossible. We know that the longer independence is maintained, the greater the quality of life that will be experienced, but the need for help and the ability to pay for the support to retain independence is balanced by the income and other resources each older person has at their disposal. Income from pensions, benefits and other insurances in old age has a direct relationship with each individual's income and education in earlier life. This affects dependence, loss and depressive mental illness (Hellström, Persson and Hallberg, 2003).

The context of each older person's ability to accommodate and explain their expectations plays a definitive part in health, adaptation to pain symptoms and access to health services. The stereotyped views of professionals on how it is to be old, and what decisions an older person should make, often affect relationships between the older person and their family members (Manthorpe, Malin and Stubbs, 2004). The holistic care of an older person in pain, based on the principles of how intrinsic or extrinsic decisions affect their independence, dignity and choice, has social and economic aspects.

References

Allen, P.F. (2005) Association between diet, social resources and oral health related quality of life in edentulous patients. *Journal of Oral Rehabilitation*, **32**, 623–8.

Auster, R., Levenson, I. and Sarachek, D. (1969) The production of health: an exploratory study. *Journal of Human Resources*, **4**, 412–36.

Barnes, M. and Bennet, G. (1998) Frail bodies, courageous voices: older people influencing community care. *Health and Social Care in the Community*, **6**(2), 102–11.

Buckley, N.J., Denton, F.T., Robb, L. and Spencer, B.G. (2004) The transition from good to poor health: an econometric study of the older population. *Journal of Health Economics*, **23**(5), 1013–34.

Byford, S., Torgerson, D. and Raftery, J. (2000) Cost of illness studies. *British Medical Journal*, **320**, 1335.

Campbell, S.E., Seymour, D.G., Primrose, W.R., Lynch, J.E., Dunstan, E., Espallargues, M., Lamura, G., Lawson, P., Philp, I. *et al.* (2005) A multi-centre European study of factors affecting the discharge destination of older people admitted to hospital: analysis of in-hospital data from the ACMEplus project. *Age and Ageing*, **34**, 467–75.

Canniscio, C., Block, J. and Kawachi, I. (2003) Social capital and successful ageing: the role of senior housing. *Annals of Internal Medicine*, **139**, 395–9.

Contoyannis, P. and Jones, A.M. (2004) Socio-economic status, health and lifestyle. *Journal of Health Economics*, **23**(5), 965–95.

Cresci, M.K. (2005) Older adults living in the community: issues in home safety. *Geriatric Nursing*, **26**(5), 282–6.

Crist, J.D. (2005) The meaning for elders of receiving family care. *Journal of Advanced Nursing*, **49**(5), 485–93.

Cully, J.A., Gfeller, J.D., Heise, R.A., Ross, M.J., Teal, C.R. and Kunik, M.E. (2005) Geriatric depression, medical diagnosis, and functional recovery during acute rehabilitation. *Archives of Physical Medicine and Rehabilitation*, **86**(12), 2256–60.

Deaton, A. (2002) Policy implications for the gradient of health and wealth. *Health Affairs*, **21**(2), 13–30.

Deaton, A. (2003) Health, inequality and economic development. *Journal of Economic Literature*, **61**, 113–58.

Department of Health (2001) *The National Service Framework for Older People*, The Stationery Office, London.

Department of Health (2005) *The Long Term (Neurological) Conditions. National Service Framework*, The Stationery Office, London.

Dickinson, A. (1999) *The food choices and eating habits of older people: a grounded theory.* Unpublished PhD thesis. Buckinghamshire and Chilterns College UK: Brunel University.

Douglas, M. (1966) *Purity and Danger. An Analysis of the Concepts of Pollution and Taboo.* Routledge, London.

Duke, D. (2006) Measuring frailty in geriatric patients. *Canadian Medical Association Journal*, **174**(3), 352. 31 January. <*http://www.cmaj.ca/cgi/content/full/174/3/352-c*> accessed on 08/03/2006.

Evans, R. (2002) Interpreting and addressing inequalities in health: from Black to Aicheson to Blair to . . . ? in, *Seventh OHE Annual Lecture. Office of Health Economics.*

Evans, R., Barer, M. and Marmor, T. (1994) *Why are Some People Healthy Andnothers Not? The Determinants of Health of Populations*, 1st edn. Walter de Gruyter, New York.

Fuchs, V.R. (2004) Reflections on the socio-economic correlates of health. *Journal of Health Economics*, **23**(4), 653–61.

Gilson, A.M., Maurer, M. and Joranson, D.E. (2005) State policy affecting pain management: recent improvements and the positive impact of regulatory health policies. *Health Policy*, **74**, 192–204.

Gomolin, I.H., Aung, M.M., Wolf-Klein, G. and Auerbach, C. (2005) Older is colder: temperature range and variation in older people. *Journal of the American Geriatrics Society*, **53**(12), 2170–2.

Gray, L. and Martin, F. (2005) Classifying patients in hospital. *Age and Ageing*, **34**, 422–4.

Guariglia, A. and Rossi, M. (2004) Private medical insurance and saving: evidence from the British Household Panel Survey. *Journal of Health Economics*, **23**(4), 761–83.

Guglielmo, W.J. (2006) Doctors: the new target in the war on drugs? *Medical Economics.* <*http://www.memag.com/memag/article/articleDetail.jsp*>

Gustafsson, K., Ekblad, J. and Sidenvall, B. (2005) Older women and dietary advice: occurrence, comprehension and compliance. *Journal of Human Nutrition and Dietetics,* **18**, 453–60.

Gustafsson, K. and Sidenvall, B. (2002) Food-related health perceptions and food habits among older women. *Journal of Advanced Nursing,* **39**, 164–73.

Gyrd-Hansen, D. (2004) Investigating the social value of health changes. *Journal of Health Economics,* **23**(6), 1101–16.

Hakamies-Blomqvist, L., Wiklund, M. and Henriksson, P. (2005) Predicting older drivers' accident involvement – Smeed's law revisited. *Accident Analysis and Prevention,* **37**, 675–80.

Hellström, Y., Persson, G. and Hallberg, I.R. (2003) Quality of life and symptoms among older people living at home. *Journal of Advanced Nursing Practice,* **48**(6), 584–93.

Hirani, V. and Primatesta, P. (2005) Vitamin D concentrations among people aged 65 years and over living in private households and institutions in England: population survey. *Age and Ageing,* **34**, 485–91.

Iversen, T. (2004) The effects of patient shortage on a general practitioners' future income and list of patients. *Journal of Health Economics,* **23**(4), 673–94.

Janlov, A-C, Hallberg, I.R. and Petersson, K. (2006) Older persons' experience of being assessed for and receiving public home help: do they have any influence over it? *Health and Social Care in the Community,* **14**(1), 26–36.

Lagergren, M. (2005) Whither care of older persons in Sweden? – a prospective analysis based upon simulation model calculations 1000–2030. *Health Policy,* **74**, 325–34.

Le Grand, J. (1991) *Equity and Choice.* Harper Collins Academic, London.

Le Grand, J. (2003) *Motivation, Agency, and Public Policy – of Knights and Knaves, Pawns and Queens.* Oxford University Press, Oxford.

Lipsitz, L.A. (2005) The elderly people of post-Soviet Ukraine: medical, social and economic challenges. *Journal of the American Geriatrics Society,* **53**(12), 2216–20.

Litaker, D. and Love, T.E. (2005) health care resource allocation and individuals' health care needs; examining the degree of fit. *Health Policy,* **73**, 183–93.

McGinnis, J. and Foege, W.H. (1993) Actual causes of death in the United States. *Journal of the American Medical Association,* **270**, 2207–12.

Manthorpe, J., Mailn, N. and Stubbs, H. (2004) Older people's views of rural life: a study of three villages. *International Journal of Older People Nursing and Journal of Clinical Nursing,* **13**(2), 97–104.

Mitnitski, A., Song, X., Skoog, I., Broe, G.A., Cox, J.L., Grunfeld, E. and Rockwood, K. (2005) Relative fitness and frailty of elderly men and women in developed countries and their relationship with mortality. *Journal of the American Geriatrics Society*, **53**(12), 2184–9.

Muira, H., Ari, Y. and Yamasaki, K. (2005) Feelings of burden and health-related quality of life among family care-givers looking after the impaired elderly. *Psychiatry and Clinical Neurosciences*, **59**, 551–5.

Muira H, Kariyasu M, Yamasaki K, Sumi Y. (2004) Physical, mental and social factors affecting self-rated verbal communication among elderly individuals. *Geriatrics, and Gerontology International*, **4**, 100–4

Nahcivan, N.O. and Demirezen, E. (2005) Depressive symptomatology among Turkish older adults with low incomes in a rural community sample. *Journal of Clinical Nursing*, **14**, 1232–40.

OECD (2001) *Aging and Transport: Mobility Needs and Safety Issues*. OECD, Paris.

Okoro, C.A., Strine, T.W., Young, S.L., Balluz, L.S. and Mokdad, A.H. (2005) Access to health care among older adults and receipt of preventive services. Results from the Behavioural Risk Factor Surveillance System 2002. *Preventive Medicine*, **40**, 337–43.

Polansky, P. and Smoyak, S. (2005) Independence, Dignity and choice in assisted living. *Journal of Psychosocial Nursing*, **43**(3), 16–19.

Pollack, C.E. and von dem Knesebeck, O. (2004) Social capital and health among the aged: comparisons between the United States and Germany. *Health and Place*, **10**, 383–91.

Roberts, K. (2001) Across the health–social care divide: elderly people as active users of health care and social care. *Health and Social Care in the Community*, **9**(2), 100–7.

Roberts, K. (2002) Issues and innovations in nursing practice. Exploring participation: Older people on discharge from hospital. *Journal of Advanced Nursing*, **40**(4), 413–20.

Schofield, P., Dunham, M., Clarke, A., Falkner, M., Ryan, T. and Howarth, A. (2005) *An Annotated Bibliography for the Management of Pain in the Older Adult*. The University of Sheffield School of Nursing and Midwifery, Sheffield.

Sheshamani, M. and Gray, A.M. (2004) A longitudinal study of the effects of age and time to death on hospital costs. *Journal of Health Economics*, **23**(2), 217–35.

Shreffler-Grant, J., Weinert, C., Nichols, E. and Ide, B. (2005) Complementary therapy use among older rural adults. *Public Health Nursing*, **22**(4), 323–31.

Smith, J.P. (1999) Healthy bodies and thick wallets: the dual relation between health and economic status. *Journal of Economic Perspectives*, **13**(2), 145–66.

Sofaer, B., Moore, A.P., Holloway, I., Lamberty, J.M., Thorpe, T.A.S. and O'Dwyer, J. (2005) Chronic pain as perceived by older people: a qualitative study. *Age and Ageing*, **34**, 462–6.

Traynor, V. (2005) Understanding the lives of older women. *Nursing Standard*, **19**(44), 41–8.

Van Hootven, C.H. and Norton, E.C. (2004) Informal care and health use of older adults. *Journal of Health Economics*, **23**(6), 1159–80.

Vincent, J.A. (2005) Understanding generations: political economy and culture in an ageing society. *The British Journal of Sociology*, **56**(4), 579–99.

Wang, H., Yip, W., Zhang, L., Wang, L. and Hsiao, W. (2005) Community based health insurance in poor rural China: the distribution of net benefits. *Health Policy and Planning*, **10**, 366–74.

'Creaking joints, a bit of arthritis, and aches and pains': older people's experiences and perceptions of pain

3

Amanda Clarke and Tony Ryan

One major area of practice development identified by older people in recent years has been the need for care practitioners to understand more fully the experience of chronic pain. Most studies concerning older people's experiences of pain use quantitative methods of inquiry. Although such approaches are helpful in describing the extent and nature of the pain experience for older people, they lack the capacity to capture a rich understanding of everyday experiences of living with chronic pain. By listening to older people describe their pain, research may help to challenge widely held beliefs about ageing, physical decline and chronic pain.

Our aim in this chapter is to contribute to a more developed understanding of pain in later life by looking at what older people themselves have to say: their experiences and perceptions of pain in the context of their everyday lives and growing older. Recent qualitative research on older people's experiences of pain, together with illustrations from Clarke's (2001) doctoral study, will be drawn on throughout the chapter.

The work around older people and chronic pain has in no way been conducted exclusively through quantitative means. A small but growing body of evidence, based on the methods of qualitative enquiry, is beginning to emerge. This evidence helps to shed light on a number of experiences associated with chronic pain. Three key themes can be identified within this literature:

- adjustment to lifestyle (Roberto and Reynolds, 2002), routines (Sofaer *et al.*, 2005) and relationships (Roberto, 2001);

- difficulties in describing and drawing attention to pain (Becker, 1999; Higgens, Madjar and Walton, 2004);

- alternative strategies for pain management (Carson and Mitchell, 1998).

In this chapter we draw attention to work that is narrative in nature, in order to further understand the experience of chronic pain.

The study

As part of her doctoral work, Clarke (2001) undertook an in-depth sociological study of the lives and views of older people aged 60–96 in the community, using a biographical approach. The main aim was to explore participants' perceptions and experiences of ageing and later life through the collection of life stories. The life stories of 'ordinary' older people (Midwinter, 1991; Hazan, 1994) were sought in the belief that, through biographical approaches, we can understand more fully the ways in which diverse experiences and attitudes throughout life, may affect individual circumstances and colour perceptions in older age (Bernard and Meade, 1993). This included exploring whether people responded to ageing in different ways, as well as what was unique and what was shared about later life.

No specific question about pain was asked; rather, people's experiences and perceptions of pain were raised spontaneously in the context of their life stories, and specifically in relation to their attitudes towards growing older. The study differed from most other studies reported here – participants were not recruited because they were suffering pain – nonetheless, the findings illuminate and add to the few reports of people's pain experiences and perceptions in their own words to be found in the pain literature (Schofield *et al.*, 2005).

Is pain different for older people?

Sanders, Donovan and Dieppe (2002) examined the meanings of symptoms for older people with severe osteoarthritis of the knee and/or hip, looking particularly at the biographical aspects (Bury, 1982, 1988) of symptoms. Older participants seemed resigned about their symptoms, portraying them as a normal and integral part of their biography and ageing. Yet they also talked about the highly disruptive impact of symptoms on their daily lives, recognizing this as abnormal. In

Clarke's study, Josephine Buxton (61) had worked as a nursing auxiliary before back pain had forced her to take early retirement. She reflected:

> As you grow older, your body changes and like infection and things like that, you don't get over them as quick as you know when you were younger. If you've got a pain, it's a different pain, it feels new, it feels like something you've never had before, you know, as I said, it takes on a different characteristic. A sore throat is not like a sore throat when you were 20 or 30, it seems to be differ- ent. And of course, one tends to get a bit slower, like you know, you put things down and you tends to mislay things and, as I was telling you, about that book, 'Where is my glasses?' You put things down and you can't find it and you feel all flustered you know and well, I can say that, I'm growing old and I'm taking things in its stages, you know, I'm lucky than most, you know, with health, touch wood.

Josephine's comments demonstrate that she felt that there is something about pain that is different in older age, as well as revealing some of the challenges this caused her in everyday life – from taking longer to get over a sore throat to mobil- ity problems caused by her back pain.

Equating older age with aches and pains

Qualitative literature suggests that older people link ageing to physical decline and being in pain (Becker, 1999; Roberto and Reynolds, 2002; Sanders, Donovan and Dieppe, 2002) therefore they may be reluctant to seek help. For example, Ross et al.'s (2002) Canadian study revealed that older people viewed moderate pain as something that needed to be lived with and therefore sought little or no profes- sional help. Similarly, Yates, Dewar and Fentiman's (1995) interviews with older Australians living in a residential setting revealed they had an expectation that they would suffer pain as they aged and therefore tended not to seek help. This is also found in the nursing-home setting where, because older people believed their pain to be intractable, they often did not complain to staff (Weiner et al., 2003, Higgens et al., 2004). Some participants in Clarke's (2001) study expressed the view that their aches and pains had to be 'put up with' since they were simply a result of ageing, a few were able to separate being ill from being old, and others acknowledged that their feelings and experiences changed from day to day (cf. Bamford, 1994; Minichiello et al., 2000). William Buxton's (79) view was typical when he said:

> As long as I've got my health and strength. As long as I've got my health, I'm all right, no pain or nothin'. I don't worry about nothin' as long as I've my health

and strength. I don't worry about having no money or anything. I don't want money, just my health and no pain . . .

Similarly, Daisy Lovett (91) commented:

I don't feel old, mentally. If I'm stiff then I think, 'Oh it must be old age'. Some days I feel pleased that I have reached that age - providing that you are well.

Like Daisy, Dipti Sur (70) related 'getting old' to 'aches and pains':

I'm getting old, but I don't feel that way; my mind is young and I want to keep it that way. I feel tired sometimes but I don't let that stop me doing things. I do have aches and pains in my joints and muscles, but I've got to do things for myself and I do them.

Betty Lomas (90) talked of 'catching up' with the physical limitations brought about by older age. She explained that she had suffered from several falls in the past year, which meant that she could not leave her flat on her own:

I had both my knees replaced when I was 58. It was wonderful, it made such a lot of difference. I feel it now, but only in stiffness, not real pain. But now I'm getting older, it's catching up a bit.

Betty's comments about her stiffness not being 'real pain' perhaps suggest that older people may trivialize their own pain as 'aches' and are reluctant to complain because they compare themselves to others who they see as worse off than themselves (see also George Daley's views below, and the section 'Managing pain'). This finding is consistent with other empirical studies (for example, Blomqvist and Edberg, 2002).

Salience of older age linked to whether people experienced pain

Participants in Clarke's (2001) study tended to associate older age with illness, pain and physical decline, whether or not they themselves were experiencing illness, pain or disability. Maureen Williams (81) felt that the experience of later life was a lot to do with attitude, 'I'm not perturbed about getting older . . . I've got a good attitude to getting older'. Maureen went on to say, however, that this could be because her health and quality of life were relatively good:

But I'm well and I'm not in pain . . . It depends on quality. If you've got no aches and pains and you have a supportive family and you've got no cares . . . In that sense, I've been blessed and am blessed. I haven't got my husband, which is dreadful, but that's [his death] two years ago now. I've been very, very fortunate and I think a lot of old people if they've got no prop at all, it must be dreadful . . .'

George Daley (78) believed that older age was partly 'a state of mind', but also that physical limitations and being in pain had an affect on whether or not he felt old. His perceptions were based on his observations of the older people he took to and from the local luncheon club every week, most of whom were disabled in some way:

The way they talk, one would think they were 20 years older, I think it is a matter of outlook partly, partly that. It is partly that, it is true that those, usually, those I carry to the luncheon club are somewhat disabled, I don't mean completely disabled but they're a bit infirm and in pain. They can't walk very far that sort of thing, um, so perhaps that needs to be taken into account, but most of them think of themselves as old, whereas I don't, I don't think of myself particularly as old, I think of myself as living. I mean not being old if you like except as I say, when I get the creaking joints occasionally and a bit of arthritis, and then you become aware, you think, 'This is part of age', but then when I'm feeling normal shall I say, when I'm not having pains or anything like that, I don't feel old, I just don't and I don't behave, I don't think as though I'm old. But I find that most of the people I talk to there do.

George Daley appeared to minimize his own 'creaking arthritic pain' in the light of the pain he witnessed from the disabled older people he drove to the local luncheon club. However, his choice of words 'when I'm feeling normal' is revealing: George did not feel old when he was free of pain, but to be in pain, to be old, made him feel different and prevented him from acting and behaving in the way he desired.

Effect of pain on everyday lives

The main foci of qualitative studies are on the effects of chronic pain on people's daily lives and their ways of adjusting and coping with chronic pain within the community setting. For example, Klinger et al. (1999) found that older people in the community adapted nearly half of their daily activities when experiencing pain, and less important tasks would be stopped altogether. This has also been noted in people with chronic pain living in nursing-home settings (Pickering *et al.*, 2001). Dickson and Kim (2003) describe a process of normalization where older women learn to 'get on with it' and develop their own management strategies. Others indicate that older people do not consider their pain to be a great problem; it was the effect pain had on their daily lives that seemed most problematic (Blomqvist and Edberg, 2002).

Participants in Clarke's (2001) study did all they could to enjoy their lives, despite their physical problems. As Thompson *et al.* (1990, p. 172) also found, 'part of the freedom of later years is to feel that if the body is ageing, the spirit is still young'. It is important, however, not to trivialize the very real physical problems that some participants experienced. Janice Roberts (64) said that she had, 'only usual aches and pains, shoulder pains, women's trouble'. She felt that this restricted her in some respects; in particular, she had given up paid work as a cleaner because of the arthritis in her shoulder. In her work as a volunteer at the RSPCA, she preferred to keep quiet about her pain:

> I know my limits, what I've got, but nobody knows about it. You know, 'Come on, give us a lift with this' and, 'Do this'. I feel so embarrassed that I sometimes do it and then I suffer after.

When Janice talked about 'what I've got', she was referring to cancer. Despite Janice's assumption that her aches and pains were a result of ageing, it was likely that she was prevented from doing all the things that she would have liked because of her condition, although this is not to say that ageing had no effect on her physical capabilities. In addition, Janice's comments that no one knew about her pain shows the disruptive effects that an 'invisible' pain may have on someone's life: they may be less likely to receive and be offered support (Hall-Lord *et al.*, 2002; Higgens, Madjar and Walton, 2004).

Violet Jones (83), had experienced a stroke and had been treated and operated on for cancer twice. Since the stroke, she had found walking painful, but she was determined that this would not affect her independence and she said that did not 'want to go yet', because, she said, 'This day and age, 83 is nothing is it?' She seemed determined not to let her pain interfere with her life:

> Not being able to walk really annoys me because people say, 'Can you walk any faster?' and I can't. All the way down on both my legs, it's pain. I'm all right sitting or driving that's fine, it's only when I walk that bothers me. Otherwise, I am very pleased to go on living and I've not ended my life with the stroke.

Since walking caused her so much pain, Violet had learnt to drive again following the stroke:

> I'm so fortunate – I did have a small stroke – I was in hospital for five weeks, so they must have thought I needed care. And when I came home, I had an automatic car but I did not know what to do with it. But the man who came was marvellous. He came five or six times and said I had only lost my confidence. He was marvellous and not bossy. He said he thought I could go on driving for another two or three years at least.

Violet had adapted to the restrictions brought about by her pain by buying an automatic car which allowed her to continue to carry out many of the activities she had always enjoyed in her life (see case study below).

Managing the pain

Blomqvist and Edberg's (2002) Swedish study undertaken with older people living in their own homes in persistent pain and receiving home care found that about half did not consider pain to be a great problem; the effect pain had on participants' daily lives seemed to be a greater problem than the pain itself. All said that pain restricted their lives, but the parts of life that were restricted differed. Blomqvist and Edberg (2002) stress the importance of ordinary everyday activities for handling pain, such as mobility and distraction. Other ways for managing pain found in the literature include: spending time with family and friends; reading and watching the television (Carson and Mitchell, 1998); rest and other interventions such as heat, massage or 'folk' remedies (Lansbury, 2000, Ross et al., 2002, Dickson and Kim, 2003); homeopathy, hot baths, salves, meditation and exercise (Roberto and Reynolds, 2002). Most studies find that medication is taken only as a last resort.

Since Clarke's study was not specially about pain, it is unsurprising that techniques for managing pain commonly found in the literature were not expressed, nor did participants discuss seeking help or receiving support from friends or relatives; however, participants did give a sense of how keeping a positive attitude, seeing others as worse off than themselves, and learning from their experiences helped them to manage their pain.

Keeping a positive attitude

Four years before her interview, Gladys Peters (93) had fallen and broken her hip. The hospital staff where she was admitted advised her to go into a nursing home, but Gladys refused:

I said, 'I know my rights and I'm not going in there, I'm not going in a home. I like my independence and I'm not'.

Instead, Gladys moved into sheltered accommodation run by the local authority. She had difficulty walking due to pain and stiffness and had not been outside by herself for nine years, but said she tried to keep a positive attitude:

I think old age is what you make it, a lot of it. I know things happen, I mean, your legs stop moving, things like that, there's nothing you can do about it, so you might as well accept it. I wake up some mornings, fresh as a daisy. Another morning, 'Oh I ache' (laughs). Funny thing, old age' (laughs).

Despite her arthritis and stiffness, and the 'final warning' served by the warden of her flat, Gladys continued to make great vats of jam on her small portable electric hob: her defiance and independence were part of her strategy to deal with her pain.

Others in relation to pain

Throughout these investigations older people reflected upon the relative nature of pain, whether it be other people's pain, or experiences in relation to themselves and their situation, how they might help or assist others or the role of other significant people in their lives.

Participants compared themselves to other older people and generally concluded that they were 'better off' than them, particularly in physical terms. Lillian Grayson (83) compared herself to the people she saw in hospital:

Sometimes when we go to the hospital and we see these people I think to meself, 'We're lucky we can walk'. We're very slow walkers now, some of these people, well I don't think I'd want to be like that.

Reginald Green (78) had lung cancer and his opinion was also shaped by his experience of visiting friends in hospital:

I'd like to be fitter than I am, but I can't grumble at my state of fitness when dear oh dear, you see some poor things in hospital. You know, one's to count one's blessings and be very, very grateful.

Maureen Williams (81) reflected:

If you're blessed with health and strength and faculties, you don't get old so young as some people get old. I mean, some people at 70 get arthritic problems, shut-in problems, pain, so it's a degree really.

Similarly, Janice Roberts (64) who had a gynaecological cancer said:

There are people that are worse than me, tons and tons, it must be terrible for them to have to wake up every day in pain and not to be able to do anything about it, I feel so sorry for them, you know, and if they can't get out, at least I can get out.

Maureen and Janice's reference to 'shut-in' problems perhaps indicate that it is only when pain affects people's everyday lives – such as not going out – that it causes a problem, and then they may seek help.

A few participants described the ways in which they used their experiences of illness to help others. Josephine Buxton (61) said:

I often say that misfortune is a process of learning to cope with life and you are able to understand what other people are going through. A lot of people if they've never experienced bad things or pain always think someone's putting it on and they have no feeling, cannot understand what's going off. But if you have suffered, you know what suffering is, what pain is, emotional pain, physical pain and psychological pain. You know what it felt like so you can help other people. And that's how I have helped other people who suffer.

Josephine's phrase 'learning to cope with life' is significant: helping others using her own experiences was one way in which Josephine could make sense of her own experiences of pain – physical and emotional – the 'misfortunes' of life.

Dorothy Twigg (82) had nursed her husband, Philip, at home when he was dying of cancer. Her account of the events leading up to her husband's diagnosis and of his death was dominated by her concerns about her husband's illness, as well as his feelings. Dorothy even referred to herself as selfish in wanting her husband to go on living since he was in a great deal of pain:

And I thought, 'Well now, I'm being selfish'. I knew I was being selfish, I was willing him to live and he was absolutely in agony. He once said to me, 'When the doctor comes, I'm going to ask him to send me into hospital'. And er, I started to cry and I said, 'Well, aren't you satisfied with what I've done?' And he said, 'Yes, I am, but it's too much for you. You're up and down here. I count the times you come upstairs.

There appears to be little in the literature about family carers and their attitude towards pain. Although Farrell *et al.* (1995) point to some of the barriers which prevent family carers from fully informing medical or health-care staff about the degree of acute pain their older parent may be experiencing, work in this area is limited and may be an avenue for further research.

Implications for practice

Caring for patients in pain is frequently central to the nurse's role (Seers, 2006) and, since older people are the largest users of health and social care services in a wide range of settings, nurses need to be able to undertake comprehensive assessments to enable older people in pain to maintain satisfactory lives. Yet this is not a simple task. Seers underlines the subjectivity, complexity and dynamic nature of pain: 'it is more than purely a result of stimulation – it includes the interaction of physical, psychological and social factors and thus each person's experience of pain is individual and unique' (Seers, 2006, p. 457). Nursing interventions to help older people in pain should therefore be based on an understanding of what it is like to live with pain, by listening to older people's accounts of their experiences and everyday lives, as we have tried to describe above. The importance of ordinary everyday activities for handling pain, such as spending time with family and friends, diversional activities, such as reading, praying and watching television (Carson and Mitchell, 1998) and rest should be stressed, as well as evaluating the effects and unwanted side effects from pain management activities (Blomqvist and Edberg, 2002). Often, medication is taken only as a last resort (Ross *et al.*, 2002). Individual plans for intervention should be compiled to manage pain by valuing older people's experiences, spending time with them and believing their complaints about pain (Blomqvist and Edberg, 2002). This can only be achieved if nurses listen to patients in order to gain a better understanding of their needs and lives.

Case studies

The following, very different, case studies are based on Clarke's research.

Abdur Rahman

Mr Rahman was born in East Pakistan (now Bangladesh). In 1962, when he was aged 25, he emigrated to England and worked in a steel moulding factory. Although he could not speak English, his work did not require language skills and he was happy there. In 1978, he suffered an accident while working on an automatic machine in the factory. His right hand and leg were badly damaged and he was taken to hospital unconscious. Mr Rahman required extensive operations to reconstruct his damaged limbs and stayed in hospital for 20 weeks. After his discharge, he spent six months as an outpatient, returning to the hospital for physiotherapy. He was lonely because his family were still living in Bangladesh: he missed his wife and three daughters. Four years after the accident, Mr Rahman's solicitors advised him to accept the small amount of compensation offered by his employers. In 1987 he brought his family to England, but by this time all his compensation money had gone.

Once he had recovered sufficiently from his injuries, Mr Rahman asked his employers if they would take him back and they agreed. After ten months, however, he was made redundant. He was not given an explanation for this but felt it was because of his disability. Since 1978 he has been unemployed, despite his efforts to obtain work. He says that employers initially accept him for work, but at the end of the day, when they see that he is not physically fit for work, they appear to change their minds. He finds this very frustrating, particularly since he is willing to accept any type of work, 'even road sweeping'.

Now aged 65, Mr Rahman reflects that this episode was the most difficult time in his life. In all, he spent four years on his own after the accident and feels that he has suffered a great deal, 'both mentally and physically'. He now spends most of his time in his small terraced house, watching television and surrounded by his family. He misses being occupied in 'something meaningful'. He rarely goes out, apart from going to the mosque, and longs for more male companionship. He describes how arthritis affects his 'every joint' which he thinks is due to older age. He also says that he has 'a lot of pain all over my body' and a stomach ulcer, which he feels, might be the result of the stress he had suffered due to the industrial accident 20 years before. In addition, he is still in severe pain from the accident and is on the NHS waiting list for further operations. He does not take his prescribed medication because he does not understand what the tablets are for. He says: 'I just want peace of mind and pray to God to give me peace'.

Violet Jones

Violet is a retired head teacher, aged 85. Her first teaching post was at a 'rough' school in the industrial east end of a northern city. Although there were 60 7-year-old pupils in Violet's class, she 'enjoyed' the experience so much that she decided that she would teach at night school too. She taught for 43 years and retired at the age of 60. She did not have the time to miss teaching: she travelled extensively around the world, staying in the US for 7 weeks.

Violet had lived with and cared for her mother until she died in her 70s. Her sister Amelia had left home when she was much younger, but if Violet wanted to go on holiday, she would occasionally come to stay. After retiring, Violet continued to live at her mother's house before moving to her present flat. A friend asked her if she would like to live with her, but Violet declined the offer: she prefers to live on her own.

Violet has difficulty walking and suffers from chronic pain in her back, hips and knees. Fourteen years ago she developed ovarian cancer, which recurred a few years later. Soon after her second treatment for cancer, Violet had a hip replacement operation, which she thought exacerbated the 'pain problem'. She stayed in hospital for five weeks and then returned home to look after herself. Soon afterwards she suffered a stroke and was again admitted to hospital for several weeks.

Violet particularly values the independence that driving gives her, but worries that she might soon have to give up because of the pain in her hips and knees – which she puts down to 'old age'. She takes medication for the pain only when it 'gets really bad' but is worried about the negative side-effects.

Violet says that she 'doesn't get bored'. She spends her week visiting and being visited by friends; sometimes they go out for a pub meal, or for a drive in the country. She has a hairdresser and a cleaner who visits her flat once a week, and she goes to a church meeting once a fortnight. She also visits two friends who are in their nineties, and helps her younger sister to her shopping. She enjoys going to the theatre, to classical music concerts and to see musicals. Recently, she has developed an interest in photography and has made her own greeting cards. Violet describes how she likes to stay 'active' and to be 'independent' and this, she feels, helps to distract her from her pain and walking problems. Nevertheless, she worries about these problems getting worse in the future and for how long she can continue caring for herself at home.

Learning point

In the following quote from Benner and Wrubel (1989), substitute the word 'illness' for pain:

[the best nursing practitioners] . . . see the patient's formal and informal nursing histories, because they know every illness has a story. Plans are threatened or thwarted, relationships are disturbed and symptoms become laden with meaning depending on what else is happening in the person's life. Understanding the meaning of the illness can facilitate treatment and cure. Even when no treatment is available and no cure is ▶

possible, understanding the meaning of illness for the person and for that person's life is a form of healing, in that such understanding can overcome the sense of alienation, loss of self-understanding, and loss of social integration that accompany illness.

Now consider:

- How might gaining a better understanding of a person's life help the nurse to recognize the complex nature of pain, including the individual's physical, psychological and social needs?
- How might the nurse sensitively respond to these needs?
- What do the case studies reveal about the potential for using ordinary everyday activities for handling pain?
- What person-centred interventions and strategies might be suggested to Mr Rahman and Miss Jones?

Summary

- **Assessment:** Nurses should focus on the individual as the definer of his or her pain experience and the strategies which help and hinder its management.
- **Planning:** Nurses should compile individual plans for intervention to manage pain by valuing older people's experiences and perceptions about their pain, and working with them and their significant others in its management.
- **Implementation:** The importance of people's ordinary, everyday activities for handling pain should not be neglected. The purpose and potential side effects of pharmacological interventions must be explained and negotiated with the individual.
- **Evaluation:** The effects and unwanted side effects from pain management activities and medication must be evaluated and discussed with the person in pain.

References

Bamford, C. (1994) *Grandparents' Lives: Men and Women in Later Life.* Age Concern Scotland, Edinburgh.

Becker, B. (1999) Narratives of pain in later life and conventions of storytelling. *Journal of Aging Studies*, **13**(1), 73–87.

Benner, R. and Wrubel, J. (1989) *The Primacy of Caring 'Stress and Coping' in Health and Illness*. Addison-Wesley, Menlo Park, CA.

Bernard, M. and Meade, K. (eds) (1993) *Women Come of Age*. Edward Arnold, London.

Blomqvist, K. and Edberg, A. (2002) Living with persistent pain: experiences of older people receiving home care. *Journal of Advanced Nursing*, **40**(3), 297–306.

Bury, M. (1982) Chronic illness as biographical disruption. *Sociology of Health and Illness*, **4**, 165–82.

Bury, M. (1988) Meaning at risk: the experience of arthritis, in *Living with Chronic Illness: The Experience of Patients and Their Families* (eds R. Anderson and M. Bury), Unwin Hyman, London.

Carson, G.M. and Mitchell, G.J. (1998) The experience of living with persistent pain. *Journal of Advanced Nursing*, **28**(6), 1242–8.

Clarke, A. (2001). *Looking back and moving forward: a biographical approach to ageing*, Thesis submitted for the degree of Doctor of Philosophy, Department of Sociological Studies, University of Sheffield.

Dickson, G.L. and Kim, J.I. (2003) Reconstructing a meaning of pain: older Korean American women's experiences with the pain of osteoarthritis. *Qualitative Health Research*, **13**(5), 675–88.

Farrell, M., Gerontol, M., Gibson, S.J. and Helme, R.D. (1995) The effect of medical status on the activity level of older pain clinic patients. *Journal of the American Geriatrics Society*, **43**(2), 102–7.

Hall-Lord, M.L., Johansson, I., Schmidt, I. and Larsson, B.W. (2002) Family members' perceptions of pain and distress related to analgesics and psychotropic drugs and quality of care of elderly nursing home residents. *Health and Social Care in the Community*, **11**(3), 262–74.

Hazan, H. (1994) *Old Age Constructions and Deconstructions*. Cambridge University Press, Cambridge.

Higgens, I., Madjar, I. and Walton, J. (2004) Chronic pain in elderly nursing home residents: the need for nursing leadership. *Journal of Nursing Management*, **12**(3), 167–73.

Klinger, L., Spaulding, S.J., Polatajko, H.J., MacKinnon, J.R. and Miller, L. (1999) Chronic pain in the elderly: occupational adaptation as a means of coping with osteoarthritis of the hip and/or knee. *Clinical Journal of Pain*, **15**(4), 275–83.

Lansbury, G. (2000) Chronic pain management: a qualitative study of elderly people's preferred coping strategies and barriers to management. *Disability and Rehabilitation*, **22**(1), 2–14.

Midwinter, E. (1991) Ten years before the mast of old age. *Generations Review*, **1**(1), 4–6.

Minichiello, V., Browne, J. and Kendig, H. (2000) Perceptions and consequences of ageism: views of older people. *Ageing and Society*, **20**(3), 253–78.

Pickering, G., Deteix, A., Eschalier, A. and Dubray, C. (2001) Impact of pain on recreational activities of nursing home residents. *Aging – Clinical and Experimental Research*, **13**(1), 44–8.

Roberto, K.A. (2001) Chronic pain and intimacy in the relationships of older adults. *Generations*, **25**(2), 65–9.

Roberto, K.A. and Reynolds, S.G. (2002) Older womens' experiences with chronic pain: daily challenges and self-care practices. *Journal of Women and Aging*, **14**(3–4), 5–23.

Ross, M., Carswell, A., Hing, M., Hollingworth, G. and Dalziel, W.B. (2001) Seniors' decision making about pain management. *Journal of Advanced Nursing*, **35**(3), 442–51.

Sanders, C., Donovan, J. and Dieppe, P. (2002) The significance and consequences of having painful and disabled joints in older age: co-existing accounts of normal and disrupted biographies. *Sociology of Health and Illness*, **24**(2), 227–53.

Schofield, P.A., Dunham, M., Clarke, A., Faulkner, M., Ryan, T. and Howarth, A. (2005) *An Annotated Bibliography for the Management of Pain in the Older Adult*. University of Sheffield, ISBN1-902411-40-4.

Seers, K. (2006) Pain and older people, in *Nursing Older People*, 4th edn (eds S. Redfern and F. Ross), pp. 457–73. Churchill Livingstone, Edinburgh.

Sofaer, B., Moore, A.P., Holloway, I., Lamberty, J.M., Thorp, T.A.S. and O'Dwyer, J. (2005) Chronic pain as perceived by older people: a qualitative study. *Age and Ageing*, **34**, 462–6.

Thompson, P., Itzin, C. and Abendstern, M. (1990) *I Don't Feel Old, the Experience of Later Life*. Oxford University Press, Oxford.

Weiner, D.K., Rudy, T.E., Glick, R.M., Boston, J.R., Lieber, S.J., Morrow, L.A. and Taylor, S. (2003) Efficacy of percutaneous electrical nerve stimulation for the treatment of chronic low back pain in older adults. *Journal of the American Geriatrics Society*, **51**(5), 599–608.

Yates, P., Dewar, A. and Fentiman, B. (1995) Pain: the views of elderly people living in long-term residential care settings. *Journal of Advanced Nursing*, **21**(4), 667–74.

Assessment of pain

4

Barry Aveyard and Pat Schofield

Introduction

In this chapter we identify and discuss issues surrounding pain assessment and the approaches to assessment that are available to us in everyday practice. We then consider some of the particular problems that may be encountered when dealing with older people, and identify some of the tools available for this group. It will be useful if you can look at the pain assessment scales that you currently use in your own area and see if you can find out where they came from or who developed them.

In September 1990 the Royal College of Surgeons and College of Anaesthetists published the report of their working party *Pain After Surgery* (RCS/RCoA, 1990; see web site listed at the end of the chapter). This report can be accessed from any library or anaesthetic department and makes recommendations regarding the management of postoperative pain in the UK. Since the report was published, many of the recommendations have been taken on board for all aspects of pain management, so it was quite a significant publication in the field of pain. One of the report's key recommendations relates to pain assessment. It suggests that assessment of pain should be recorded by the nurse along with other routine observations of blood pressure and pulse. This recommendation has been adopted in many areas of health care, and many trusts now have pain assessment charts that are incorporated into their observation charts.

Before discussing pain assessment in older adults, we need to look at the issues around pain assessment in general. So in this first section we look at the history and development of pain assessment in practice. This is followed by a section focusing on assessment in older adults with and without cognitive impairment, and finally we discuss assessment for older adults in terminal care.

The need for pain assessment

Learning point

Can you think of some reasons why it is important to carry out a formal pain assessment?

You will have probably identified some of the following reasons:

- **Professional accountability.** It is a NMC requirement that all registered nurses maintain their records, and documentation errors can result is disciplinary hearings.
- **Legal requirement.** Legal judgements have found people guilty of negligence where pain assessment has not been documented within the medical or nurses' notes (Shapiro, 1994). If assessment has not been carried out, then pain management may well not be effective. As highlighted previously, the Royal College of Surgeons suggest that assessment is the start of the process of pain management and therefore fundamental to effective care.
- **Patients' reassurance.** If we talk to patients in an open and honest way about their pain then they will feel more relaxed and in control, which will help them to cope better.
- **Faster recovery.** By assessing pain we are more likely to treat it more effectively, which in turn improves care and subsequently recovery.
- **Formal record.** By presenting a formal, evidence-based record of our assessment of pain we are more likely to convince other members of the multidisciplinary team of the need for intervention and to highlight when approaches are not working.
- **Improved understanding.** By using an assessment we are able to determine which approaches are effective and which are not, and this will help us to be more creative and innovative in our approaches to pain management.

Before we can begin our assessment, there are two factors that must be taken into consideration:

- The approach to assessment must be adapted to the clinical situation. It would be unrealistic to spend hours completing lengthy pain assessment charts in a busy A&E department where the priority of care is to save lives.

- The type of pain is also an important consideration: is it acute, chronic or cancer pain? A person in acute pain will not be able to give detailed information but will be more concerned about pain relief – think of a patient coming into A&E following major trauma! In contrast, someone with chronic pain will be prepared to discuss their pain in more detail and so this assessment will be more complex and comprehensive. A cancer patient may tire easily, so again our assessment may need to be adapted.

The key issue is to be flexible. We need to be aware of the whole range of pain tools that are available and adapt them to suit our situation and our particular patient/client group.

Learning point

Take a look at Chapter 6 and remind yourself of the differences between acute and chronic pain

Before any pain assessment can be carried out, there are certain points that need to be addressed:

- onset
- pattern
- quality
- relieves
- improves
- treatments
- understanding
- intensity
- goals.

These are all important, but if the person is severe pain we need to deal with it immediately and then come back and ask these questions when they are more comfortable. The most important issue is **intensity**, and this is the aspect that we will come back to when we evaluate treatment.

Measuring the intensity of pain

Several measures are available to measure pain intensity.

Visual analogue scale (Figure 4.1a)

The visual analogue scale (VAS) is a 10 cm line with 'no pain' at one end and 'worst pain imaginable' at the other. The patient is asked to rate the level of pain that they are currently experiencing. The end-point descriptors should not be changed.

The VAS can be completed by children as young as five all the way through the age spectrum to older adults. Occasionally, some may find it confusing and so explanation is important .

Numerical rating scale (Figure 4.1b)

This is a visual analogue scale with numbered ratings along the line. These can be either 0–10 or 0–5. It is similar to the VAS in terms of suitability for a wide age range, in fact it has been suggested that older adults cope well with this measure, but we will come back to this later in the chapter. The danger is that patients tend to put a mark near to the number as opposed to a true reading, which can be misleading. This is important particularly in research terms when pain changes, even minimal changes are highly relevant.

Verbal descriptors

This scale consists of a number of labelled boxes that can be ticked by the patient or member of staff. The problem with this scale is that patients can sometimes comment that their pain is worse than moderate but not quite severe. Also, in some areas, extra boxes have been added which detracts from the validity of the tool as this amended format has not been validated.

(a) Visual analogue scale

No pain_____Worst pain imaginable

(b) Numerical rating scale

0_____1_____2_____3_____4_____5_____6_____7_____8_____9_____10

Figure 4.1   (a) Visual analogue scale. (b) Numerical rating scale

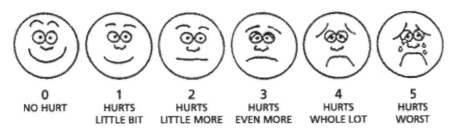

Figure 4.2   The faces pain scal

Faces pain scale *(Figure 4.2)*

This was first introduced for children, as it was found that they could relate to the expressions on the faces in terms of how they were feeling (Bieri *et al.*, 1990). It has since been found that some adults also prefer this tool.

Colour scale

This is also based on the VAS and uses colour to indicate increasing severity of the pain. Thus red is associated with really severe pain, and green/blue represents none to mild pain.

McGill Pain Questionnaire (MPQ)

The McGill Pain Questionnaire (MPQ) is a very important pain measure. Developed by Melzack and Torgerson (1975) it was designed to measure the quality of pain. The investigators carried out research to identify descriptors that are used by people to describe their pain. They then tested these descriptors and refined them to form the tool. The questionnaire now contains 78 descriptors and has been translated into 18 languages for cross-cultural use. It is a reliable and valid measure of pain quality. This is a useful tool often used in the field of chronic pain and has been used in children as young as five, right through to older adults. Although it only takes five minutes to complete and five minutes to analyse, many practitioners find it too complicated for everyday use. However, it is useful for patients who are unable to describe their pain as it can help them to put it into words.

Learning point

- Think of a time when you last experienced pain – what words would you use to describe it? Not easy, is it?

- Looking at the McGill scale – are any of your 'pain descriptors' on the list?
- Now going back to your pain assessment tool – how do you think it rates, compared to the tools discussed above?
- Are you happy that your tool is evidenced based and has not been adapted?
- Would you consider a more appropriate tool?
- Can you identify groups of patients that would not be able to complete any of these scales?

Pain assessment in patients with communication problems

We now consider pain assessment tools for those groups who perhaps have communications problems.

Although we should try to avoid using stereotypes when considering which older people may experience communication problems, there are some groups of older people for whom the challenges may be considerable. These groups may include in particular:

- older people with sensory impairment;
- older people with a learning disability;
- older people with a cognitive impairment.

In this section we consider each of these areas in more detail, with a specific focus on what might be the impact on the lives of older people.

Sensory impairment

When thinking about sensory impairment, it is only too easy to just to think that we are considering the needs of people who are blind or deaf. This can be misleading, in that for many people being blind does not mean having no sight at all, and being deaf does not mean always having no hearing. Generally, the reality is that sight or hearing is reduced. It is very easy to apply the labels 'blind' or 'deaf' without fully understanding what these terms mean for the individual patient. The reality is that there is a difference between being blind and having no sight, or being deaf and having no hearing. This is important, and we need to have clear knowledge of the true extent of the individual's disability, so that we can respond appropriately.

It is also important to use simple interventions, such as always ensuring that people who wear glasses have access to them, and people who use hearing aids are able to wear them when they want. These very basic interventions enable a more effective pain assessment by involving the person in the process.

It is usually the case that the person we are caring for is the expert in their own pain and we should be guided by them as to the best way to provide support. This again may be key to the provision of quality pain assessment.

Learning point

What might be the challenges of assessing pain when a person has a sensory impairment?

Learning disability

As people in general are living longer, so too are people with a learning disability and therefore, there is a likelihood that we will see more pain in this group. Older people with a learning disability are probably a group that is very much ignored by society (Thompson and Wright 2001). They are often cared for in inappropriate care environments by staff who do not have expertise in the field.

Donovan (2002) suggested that although nurses qualified in the area of learning disability nursing demonstrate good skills in the assessment of pain amongst this population, nurses who not experienced in this field tend to have more problems in carrying out good-quality pain assessment.

Learning point

What do you think could be the reasons for this?

Kerr, Cunningham and Wilkinson (2006) suggest that a key element in effective management of pain in older people with learning disabilities is to talk to them as individuals and listen to their experiences of pain. This is an area of health care where there is a case for good interprofessional working and well-established lines of communication. Health-care professionals who are not experienced in the field of learning disability need to be able to access support and advice when needed. If this support is not available then it is clear that staff may encounter difficulties: wanting to ensure that they manage pain effectively, but lacking the appropriate experience, they fail to carry out a clear comprehensive pain assessment.

A range of potential pain assessment tools, and the importance of being able to use a tool appropriate for the individual patient, have been discussed earlier in this chapter. It is important to emphasize this point in the area of learning disability. The use of a standard tool across a particular area will not always work; it is much more effective to choose a tool appropriate to individual. It is also important to ensure that the tool chosen is based on a knowledge of the abilities of the individual patient. It can be very tempting to assume that the best assessment tool for an older person with a learning disability might be a tool such as the faces pain scale (see Figure 4.2). However, this may involve making numerous assumptions about the person's abilities just because they have a learning disability, rather than taking time to get to know them as a person and be clear about their level of ability rather than disability.

Cognitive impairment

When considering cognitive impairment and older people it is often tempting to think immediately about dementia. Although around 750,000 people in the UK experience some degree of dementia (Alzheimer's Society, 2006), the reality is that most older people do not have dementia. Therefore it is important to recognize the importance of good-quality assessment and history-taking to obtain a clear and accurate picture of the mental ability of the individual.

Other significant causes of cognitive impairment that must not be overlooked when encountering a confused older person include:

- infection
- metabolic disorders
- hypoxia
- endocrine disorders
- drug reactions/interactions.

A key indicator that cognitive impairment may be the result of delirium rather than dementia is the nature of its onset. Delirium tends to develop rapidly over a space of hours or days at the very most, whereas most types of dementia have a much more insidious onset and develop more slowly.

There are around 60 differing types of dementia, with Alzheimer's disease being the most prevalent (Alzheimer's Society, 2006). Increasingly, just using the term dementia as a diagnosis is seen as unacceptable, as the differing diseases have unique elements and respond to interventions in differing ways. For instance,

cognitive-enhancing drugs such as donepezil (Aricept), which can
enhanced cognitive abilities for a person with Alzheimer's disease, are n
priate for a person with vascular dementia.

Perception of pain

When considering pain assessment and cognitive impairment it is important to
take several issues into account. Some researchers have implied that the ability
of people with advanced dementia to experience pain is diminished because of the
deterioration of the neurological pathways within the brain. (Blennow, 1993)
Others have suggested that this is a naive view of the situation, and that people
with dementia do not have any reduction in their experience of pain: the reality
is that they have an impaired ability to communicate their experiences of pain.
(Ferrell, 1996).

Many staff perceive agitated or difficult behaviour as a significant day-to-day
challenge in dementia care. They may also believe that this type of behaviour has
a direct link with the neurological deterioration of the brain. However, as Kitwood
(1997) clearly stated, all behaviour in dementia is an attempt to communicate.
Taking this point on board may be very significant in attempting to understand
how a person with dementia may attempt to communicate their experience of
pain.

Learning point

How might a person with dementia behave if they are experiencing pain?

It is vitally important that nurses, wherever they are working, attempt to
develop an understanding of the needs of people with dementia. If they do not,
the consequences for the person can be very serious, as has been demonstrated
when pain has become a medical catastrophe before it has been diagnosed.

If a person is seen as agitated, and their behaviour as challenging and difficult, it would be very easy to assume that the use of sedative medication is the
best way to manage the situation. However, there are real problems with the use
of sedation in the care of people with dementia. Although there may be a role
for the use of medication such as haloperidol if a person is showing signs of
true aggression, there is no real evidence that such medication will have any
impact on agitated behaviour (Lonergan *et al.*, 2002). Sedation may well lead
to an increase in agitation, and make the person more vulnerable to falling
(Alzheimer's Scotland, 2001).

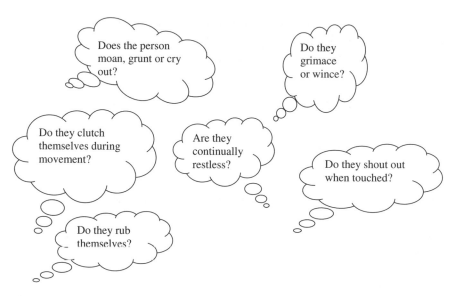

Figure 4.3 Pain behaviours

Research studies have suggested that care staff and nurses sometimes have problems in making the connection between so-called 'problem behaviour' and pain experience of a person with dementia (Sherder and van Manen, 2004). The complexity of ensuring good-quality pain assessment in dementia care has been clearly articulated (Brummel-Smith *et al.*, 2002).

The pain assessment tools discussed earlier in the chapter can have value in the assessment of pain in dementia care, and their use should always be considered. It is all too easy to assume that because a person has dementia they will not be able to respond to traditional pain assessment tools. However, some people with dementia do indeed have difficulty responding to these tools. The importance of observation of behaviours then becomes of vital importance. Horgan (2003) advocates the use of the checklist for non-verbal behaviours, (Feldt, 2000), which involves thinking whether the person expresses any of the behaviours listed in Figure 4.3. Such behaviours have been incorporated into behavioural pain assessment tools by many authors.

Behavioural pain assessment tools

A recent literature review identified 42 articles related to pain assessment, of which 10 papers particularly focused on pain in adults with cognitive impairment and 9 discussed the development of specific scales for this group. It is important to note, however, that the literature suggests that for most older adults with mild to moderate cognitive impairment, verbal report of pain can be used as a reliable indicator, just as it can with older adults who are not cognitively impaired (Kaasalainen and Crook, 2004). This suggests that specific behavioural tools are only necessary for use with adults who are severely cognitively impaired.

DS-DAT scale

One of the early and much quoted papers demonstrating the development of a pain assessment tool is that of Hurley et al. (1992). This American paper presents the results of a study developing a tool specifically for patients with advanced dementia of the Alzheimer type (DS-DAT). The initial study generated the content domain for the DS-DAT by conducting semi-structured interviews with staff in Alzheimer centres. The investigators were able to produce a list of 26 behaviours that were believed to manifest discomfort in this group of patients and 18 key signs were identified. The investigators also conducted a longitudinal study to examine the internal consistency of the scale in 82 residents.

The authors concluded that the scale was useful for the evaluation of 'comfort promoting interventions' (p. 375). Although it was a promising development, sadly, no further evidence of testing of this scale could be found in the literature. Furthermore, no rating scale was applied and so the scale became merely a checklist of behaviours. Nevertheless, many other scale developers have used the DS-DAT as a basis for the development of their own scales

Checklist of non-verbal pain indicators (CNPI)

A few years later Feldt (2000) proposed the checklist of non-verbal pain indicators (CNPI). This tool was developed following an extensive review of the literature and adding to the University of Alabama Birmingham Pain Behaviour Scale (UAB-PBS) from which the author eliminated four pain behaviours.

The instrument is designed to measure pain behaviours in cognitively impaired older adults and was tested in a pilot study of 88 cognitively impaired and cognitively intact hip fracture patients, most of whom (86%) were female. Behaviours were correlated with self-report of pain and of the six behaviours identified, facial grimaces/winces occurred in 44% of the patients tested. The investigators acknowledge that this was a very small part of a larger study and planned to evaluate further. Also, this study was conducted in an acute pain setting and further study would be required to validate the tool in a chronic pain setting.

ADD protocol

This tool, also developed in the USA, consists of a protocol that was designed to assess several factors:

- Discomfort in people who can no longer describe their pain.
- Accurate and thorough treatment of physical discomfort.
- Decreased inappropriate use of psychotropic medication.

The project described by Kovach *et al.* (1999) was one aspect of a larger educational study designed to improve pain management practice. Fifty-seven long-term care facilities were recruited into the study and an education strategy was introduced over a period of 12 months which included the addition of the Assessment of Discomfort in Dementia (ADD) protocol. Thirty-two volunteer nurses from 25 of the facilities agreed to participate in a pilot assessment of the utility of the ADD, which had been developed following a review of the literature and an adaptation of the DS-DAT scale.

Evaluation of the protocol identified a number of problems, including time, resistance to change and lack of education regarding the use of the protocol. Positive comments included an increased staff awareness of residents' discomfort; 44% commented that they found it helpful. The authors concluded that the protocol was useful and recommended further evaluation using randomized controlled trials. However, further studies have not so far been identified within the literature.

DOLOPLUS scale

In 1995 a group known as DOLOPLUS was formed to evaluate a scale designed to measure pain in the non-communicative elderly, developed from work with children (Wary, 2001). The group refined the scale which was later released as DOLOPLUS-2 and consists of 10 items organized into 3 subgroups; somatic, psychomotor and psychosocial. Each is rated according to level of intensity (0–3), thus providing an overall score of 0–30.

Test – retest validity, concurrent validity and inter-rater reliability were evaluated in a series of studies in France and Switzerland in which the authors report positive outcomes (Lefebre-Chapiro and the DOLOPLUS group, 2001). But further validation testing will need to be carried out on an international level before the tool can be accepted, and reliability will also need to be further assessed. On a pragmatic level, the DOLOPLUS-2 has been reported within the UK as being rather complex for staff within the care-home setting to complete. Further investigation would be required to confirm this anecdotal evidence.

The NOPAIN scale

The NOPAIN scale (non-communicative patient's pain assessment instrument) (Snow *et al.*, 2001) was developed following observation of behaviours while carrying out activities of living such as bathing and dressing. The tool is divided into four main sections:

1 The caregiver is asked to provide information regarding the care being delivered at the time of assessment.

2 The next section provides the carer with six pain behaviours (words, noises, faces, rubbing, bracing, restlessness).

3 The carer is asked to state if these behaviours were identified and score them on an intensity scale of 1–5.

4 The carer is asked to rate the overall pain intensity for the day using a pain thermometer.

The tool was evaluated in two studies with trained and untrained staff in care homes in the USA. There is evidence of moderate validity and reliability testing, but content validation will be required. The items identified within this scale do not appear to be generated conceptually, but they reflect those identified by Feldt (1998).

Pain assessment scale for dementing elderly (PADE)

Villaneuva *et al.* (2003) later developed the Pain Assessment Scale for Dementing Elderly (PADE). Again this scale was developed in the USA and was designed to help carers determine the presence of pain in residents of care homes. Twenty-four items were identified, in three parts, on the basis of a literature review, and interviews and observations with care-home staff. The items were categorized into three main themes and validated in three clinical settings. Reliability and validity were assessed by evaluation of the scale in a number of long-term care settings with residents suffering from dementia, but much further investigation is needed before this tool can be accepted. There is little evidence to support the credibility of the behaviours as determined by the unqualified carers, and the validation panels were not clearly identified as being separate from the study.

PAINAD

This scale was developed in the USA to assess pain in people with advanced dementia (Warden, Hurley and Volicer, 2003). It was developed using a combination of expert clinicians and observational methods. The literature review by the authors recognized the DS-DAT scale, but they commented that this scale was too complicated and therefore based their scale on the FLACC (The Face, Legs, Activity, Cry and Consolability) scale which is used with children (Merkel, Voepel-Lewis and Malviya, 2002). Initially, the scale was rated by the investigator, three trained nurses and two untrained carers. Later the psychometric properties of the scale were examined using an expert panel of nurses and a social worker from the dementia special care unit where the study was carried out. Observations of the residents were then carried out and the scale used and compared against the DS-DAT scale. The investigators reported adequate evidence of inter-rater reliability and construct validity but the sample size was very small – only 19 residents and 6 staff – so further work will need to be done on this scale. Nevertheless it is less complex than the DS-DAT scale and therefore easier for staff to administer, although the authors commented that training for use of this scale required a few hours, which is an important consideration in practical settings.

PACSLAC

A further scale developed in Canada is the PACSLAC (Pain Assessment Checklist for Seniors with Limited Ability to Communicate) (Fuchs-Lacelle and Hadjistavro-poulis, 2004). This study was conducted in three phases. Phase 1 involved the investigators conducting interviews with experienced nurses and care assistants to generate a list of behaviours; in phase 2 the nurses were asked to complete the checklist whilst carrying out potentially pain-provoking procedures; and phase 3 involved an evaluation of the scale in terms of determining pain events. Twenty-eight staff were involved in the first phase of the study, with 40 registered nurses taking part in phase 2. Residents were not actively involved in the study but they were assessed by staff using the scale in phases 2 and 3. Upon completion of the three phases, the authors concluded that the scale was easy to complete and could be completed within 5 minutes, thus concluding that there is a potential for use of this scale within long-term care facilities. However, the caregivers were asked to provide retrospective reports of the pain, which could be influenced by memory bias, and although the psychometric properties of the scale were deemed to be good, further multicentre studies would need to be carried out. The scale appears on face value to be fairly complicated, so again there are important training issues.

Abbey scale

The final scale reviewed here is that of Abbey et al. (2004) which was reported in a two-stage Australian study. The study was designed to develop a highly reliable pain scale for people with end-stage dementia and was carried out in 24 residential care facilities across 4 states. Initially 12 pain measures were identified, which were then refined to leave the scale with 6. Each of the 6 items was given a potential score of 3 grades (0–2, 3–7, 8–13), so a score of 18 indicates very severe pain. Staff were then asked to complete the scale independently for each resident, thus confirming inter-rater reliability. Facilities that were included in the first stage were again asked to participate in this second stage, and new facilities were also added. Uniquely to this study, qualitative evidence relating to their views of the scale was also collected from staff. The authors conclude that they have demonstrated evidence of reliability and validity, but they acknowledge that depression, fatigue and agitation can confound their behaviours. In spite of this the scale is easy to administer, which is an important issue when working in busy care settings. However, further reliability and validity testing will need to be carried out.

A paper published recently in the USA has reviewed all of the behavioural scales and recommends guidelines for pain assessment in this group.

Although assessment of behaviours is not always fail-safe, it can provide an excellent indicator that a person may be experiencing pain or discomfort. However, as with all assessment it cannot and must not be a one-off activity; it needs to be done frequently, in an attempt to evaluate the impact of any pain management. It is clearly not appropriate to assume that any pain management intervention will have been effective, and therefore there is no need to reassess pain. It is important to remember that the person may not be able to verbally confirm that the intervention has controlled the pain, so re-assessment is vital.

There are some formal dementia care assessment tools such as Dementia Care Mapping (Kitwood and Bredin, 1992) or the Positive Response Schedule (Perrin, 1997). These tools are comprehensive in their ability to assess the total well-being of people with dementia; they are observational tools which use a scoring system to identify signs of well-being and ill-being in the person with dementia. Both these tools can provide very detailed information about the individual and the relationship they have with the person caring for them. They may have a significant impact on the ability to identify chronic pain particularly, as they involve detailed observation over a period of time. However, they both need to be carried out by people who are experienced in their use. They therefore have limited application and are possibly more useful in dedicated dementia care areas rather than more acute areas such as medical wards that are caring for people with dementia.

Assessment of pain in terminal care

A recent review of the literature revealed 31 papers relating to this aspect of pain assessment. Many of the papers reported that pain assessment in terminal care is generally inadequate and suggest further education of staff in order to make improvements.

However, it is interesting to note that one of the problems highlighted is that in terminal care assessment of pain intensity alone is not adequate. The authors recommend a more holistic approach to assessment which includes quality of life (Schofield et al. 2006). Some of the studies incorporated quality of life measures into their assessment protocols, for example the EORTC, although the general conclusion was that further development and testing of these scales was also needed. It was particularly interesting to note that one author (Schofield *et al.* 2006) highlighted specific issues such as gender as having a significant impact upon pain intensity. The studies seem to suggest that assessment protocols should be incorporated into practice to address these issues. Hence a multimodal approach to pain assessment should be introduced.

Another important finding was that more experienced nurses are better at pain assessment, which is often the opposite of the situation in traditional settings where it has been suggested that empathy with pain decreases with years qualified.

Many of the studies used the Brief Pain Inventory (BPI) as a measure of pain assessment. This tool is becoming popular in many areas of health care; for example, the Residential Brief Pain Inventory developed in Australia. The review of the literature appears to suggest that the BPI applies well to palliative care settings, although there is a suggestion that it needs to be validated more widely across cultures. For example, Saxena, Mendoza and Cleeland (1999) point out that in India there needs to be more development of pain assessment tools. Simply translating western assessment tools into other languages does not ensure cultural sensitivity; assessment tools must be designed to meet the needs of individual cultures. This finding is supported by Chung, Wong and Yang (2000) who highlighted that Chinese cultural beliefs clearly impact upon responses to pain, and therefore pain assessment tools must be developed which respond to these beliefs. Other scales that are effective in terminal care include the visual analogue scale, numerical rating scale, verbal rating scale and the McGill Pain Questionnaire.

The final issue highlighted in this literature review relates to the timing of pain assessment. It is apparent that as the disease progresses pain assessment becomes less effective, particularly towards the end stage of the illness.

Conclusion

This chapter has attempted to articulate the vital importance of careful, good-quality pain assessment in the care of older people. We have emphasized that this can be very complex when working with older people who experience a range of communication problems.

The literature suggests that traditional pain assessment tools can be used with older adults with mild to moderate levels of dementia. However, where this is not possible, behavioural indicators can provide reliable signs of the existence of pain and should be used as a good indicator of the presence of pain. A range of behavioural tools exist and although they require further research to support their use, it is interesting to note that they are generally consistent in the behaviours that they all consider to be representative of pain (Table 4.1).

Table 4.1 Pain behaviours identified by authors

Hurley et al.	Feldt	Kovach et al.	Wary and DOLOPLUS group	Snow et al.	Villanueva et al.	Warden et al.	Fuchs-Lacelle and Hadjistavropoulis	Abbey et al.
DS-DAT	CHPI	ADD	DOLOPLUS	NOPAIN	PADE	PAINAD	PACSLAC	Abbey
Noisy breathing	Non-verbal vocalizations	Tense body language and repetitive movement	Somatic complaints	Words	Facial expression	Breathing	Activity/body movement	Vocalization
Negative vocalization	Facial grimacing	Fidgeting	Body posture	Noises	Breathing pattern	Negative vocalization	Facial expression	Facial expression
Content facial expression	Bracing	Physical aggression	Protection of sore areas	Faces	Posture	Facial expression	Vocal behaviours	Body language
Sad facial expression	Rubbing	Tearfulness	Expression	Rubbing	Proxy evaluation of pain	Body language	Social personality mood	Behavioural changes
Frightened facial expression	Restlessness	Delusions	Sleep patterns	Bracing	Dressing	Consolability	Eating, sleeping	Physiological changes

Table 4.1 Continued

Hurley et al.	Feldt	Kovach et al.	Wary and DOLOPLUS group	Snow et al.	Villaneuva et al.	Warden et al.	Fuchs-Lacelle and Hadjistavropoulis	Abbey et al.
Frown	Vocal complaints	Withdrawal behaviour	Washing/dressing	Restlessness	Feeding			Physical changes
Relaxed body language		Sad or frightened facial expression	Mobility		Transfer			
Tense body language		Verbal outburst	Communication					
Fidgeting		Repetitive waking at night	Social life					
		Phobias or fears	Behaviour problems					
		Hallucinations						
		Noisy breathing						

A key message of the chapter is that pain assessment must be individualized and appropriate to the needs of the person. It is important to recognize that there will be inevitable difficulties if a ward or unit tries to develop an assessment tool that is applied without discretion to all patients. There must be an approach to pain assessment that ensures the use of a variety of assessment methods so that a tool can be selected that best meets the needs of individual patients or clients. Finally, if the staff feel that pain is present, it is important not to ignore its existence as this can be detrimental to the health and well-being of the older adult. Remember: 'Pain management is a basic human right and failure to relieve pain is morally and ethically unacceptable' (RCS/RCoA, 1990).

References

Abbey, J., Piller, N., DeBellis, A., Esterman, A., Parker, D. and Giles, L. (2004) The Abbey pain scale: a 1-minute numerical indicator for people with end stage dementia. *International Journal of Palliative Nursing*, **10**(1), 6–13.

Alzheimer's Scotland (2001) *Drugs Used During Dementia*. Alzheimer's Scotland, Edinburgh.

Alzheimer's Society (2006) *Position Statement on Demography*. Available at: <*http://www.alzheimers.org.uk/News_and_Campaigns/Policy_Watch/demography.htm*>

Bieri, D., Reeve, R.A., Champion, G.D., Addicoat, L. and Zeigler, J.B. (1990) The faces scale for the self assessment of the severity of pain experienced by children: development, initial validation and preliminary investigation for ratio scale properties. *Pain*, **41**, 139–50.

Blennow, K. (1993) Low frequency of post lumbar headache in demented patients. *Neurologica Scandinavia*, **88**(3), 221–3.

Brummel-Smith, K., London, M.R., Drew, N., Krulewitch, H., Singer, C. and Hanson, L. (2002) Outcomes of pain in frail older adults with dementia. *Journal of the American Geriatrics Society*, **50**, 1847–51.

Chung, J.W.Y., Wong, T.K.S. and Yang, J.C.S. (2000) The lens model assessment of cancer pain. *Cancer Nursing*, **23**(6), 454–61.

Donovan, J. (2002) Learning disability nurses' experiences of being with clients who may be in pain. *Journal of Advanced Nursing*, **38**(5), 458–66.

Ferrell, M. (1996) The impact of dementia on the pain experience. *Pain*, **67**(1), 7–15.

Feldt, K.S. (2000) The checklist on nonverbal pain indicators (CNPI) *Pain Management Nursing*, **1**(1), 13–21.

Fuchs-Lacelle, S. and Hadjistavropoulis, T. (2004) Development and preliminary validation of the pain assessment checklist for seniors with limited ability to communicate (PACSLAC). *Pain Management Nursing*, **5**(1), 1–19.

Horgas, A.L. (2003) Pain management in elderly adults. *Journal of Infusion Nursing,* **26**(3), 161–5.

Hurley, A.C., Volicer, B.J., Hanrahan, P.A., Houde, S. and Volicer, L. (1992) Assessment of discomfort in advanced Alzheimer patients. *Research in Nursing and Health,* **15**, 369–77.

Kaasalainen, S. and Crook, J. (2004) An exploration of seniors' ability to report pain. *Clinical Nursing Research,* **13**(3), 199–215.

Kerr, D., Cunningham, C. and Wilkinson, H. (2006) *Responding to the Pain Experiences of People with a Learning Difficulty and Dementia.* Joseph Rowntree Foundation, York.

Kitwood, T. (1997) *Dementia Reconsidered.* Open University Press, Buckingham.

Kitwood, T. and Bredin, K. (1992) A new approach to the evaluation of dementia care. *Journal of Advances in Health and Nursing Care,* **1**, 41–60.

Kovach, Cr., Weissman, D.E., Griffie, J., Matsn, S. and Muchka, S. (1999) Assessment and treatment of discomfort for people with late stage dementia. *Journal of Pain and Symptom Management,* **18**(6), 1–11.

Lefebre-Chapiro, S. and the DOLOPLUS group (2001) The DOLOPLUS-2 scale – evaluating pain in the elderly. *European Journal of Palliative Care,* **8**(5), 191–4.

Lonergan, E., Luxenberg, J., Colford, J. and Birks, J. (2002) Haloperidol for agitation in dementia. *Cochrane Review,* **2**.

Melzack, R. and Torgerson, W.S. (1975) On the language of pain. *Anaesthesiology,* **34**, 50–90.

Merkel, S., Voepel-Lewis, T. and Malviya, S. (2002) Pain assessment in infants and young children: the FLACC scale: a behavioural tool to measure pain in young children. *American Journal of Nursing,* **102**(10), 55–8.

Perrin, T. (1997) The Positive Response Schedule for severe dementia. *Aging and Mental Health,* **1**(2), 184–91.

RCS/RCoA (1990) *Pain after Surgery.* Royal College of Surgeons and College of Anaesthetists HMSO, London.

Saxena, A., Mendoza, T. and Cleeland, C.S. (1999) The assessment of cancer pain in North India: the validation of the Hindi brief pain inventory –BPI-H. *Journal of Pain and Symptom Management,* **17**(1), 27–41.

Schofield, Smith, Clarke, Faulkner, Ryan, Kirshbaum, Aveyard, Dunham, Gell, Steele, Keogh (2006) *An Annotated Bibliography for Pain Relief in the Terminal Stages of Palliative Care.* University of Sheffield.

Shapiro, R.S. (1994) Liability issues in the management of pain. *Journal of Pain Symptoms and Management,* **9**(3), 146–52.

Sherder, E. and van Manen, F. (2004) Pain in Alzheimer's disease: nursing assistants' and Patients' evaluations. *Journal of Advanced Nursing,* **52**(2), 151–8.

Snow, A.L., Weber, J.B. and O'Malley, K.J. (2004) NOPAIN: a nursing assistant administered pain assessment instrument for use in dementia, *Dementia Geriatric Cognitive Disorders,* **17**, 240–6.

Thompson, D. and Wright, S. (2001) *Misplaced and Forgotten: People with Learning Disabilities in Residential Services for Older People.* The Mental Health Foundation, London.

Villaneuva, M.R., Smith, T.L., Erickson, J.S., Lee, A.C. and Singer, C.M. (2003) Pain assessment for the dementing elderly (PADE) Reliability and validity of a new measure. *Journal of the American Medical Directors Association,* **4**, 1–8.

Warden, V., Hurley, A.C. and Volicer, L. (2003) Development and psychometric evaluation of the pain assessment in advanced dementia scale (PAINAD). *Journal of the American Medical Directors Association,* **Feb**, 9–15.

Wary, B. (2001) Using DOLOPLUS for measuring pain among non-verbal or cognitively impaired elderly patients. *Written Communication,* **19**, 25–127.

Web sites

Australian Pain Society report, *Pain in Residential Aged Care Facilities – Management Strategies*: <*http://www.apsoc.org.au/owner/files/9e2c2n.pdf*>

British Pain Society: <*http://www.britishpainsociety.org/*>

European Federation of IASP Chapters (EFIC): <*http://www.efic.org/*>

International Association for the Study of Pain (IASP): <*http://www.iasp-pain.org/index.html*>

Patient UK Dementia: <*http://www.patient.co.uk/showdoc/23068719/*>

Royal College of Surgeons of England, *Report of the Working Party on Pain After Surgery*: <*http://www.rcseng.ac.uk/rcseng/content/publications/docs/pain_after_surgery.html*>

Communication and pain

5

David Reid

Introduction

> The word 'communicate' is historically related to the word 'common'. It stems from the Latin verb *communicare*, which means 'to share', 'to make common', and which in turn is related to the Latin word for common: *communis*. When we communicate, we make things common. We thus increase our shared knowledge, our 'common sense' — the basic precondition for all community (Rosengren, 2000).

Pain is not necessarily an accompaniment to older age, and not all older people have a disability that impedes communication. However, for those with a form of dementia (5% of 65 year olds to 20% of 85 year olds (Hofman *et al.*, 1991)) who experience pain there are clearly pressing reasons for health professionals to pay attention to communication.

What do people with dementia experience? 'What does their condition mean to them?' (Binstock, 1992). Within the academic community the 'experience of dementia' is a topic of theoretical debate (e.g. Bender and Cheston, 1997; Kitwood, 1997a; Woods, 2001) and the focus of empirical research. An indication of the importance attached to both the experience of dementia and its investigation through research activity is seen in some of the recent substantive areas of interest. The subjective experience of people with dementia has been sought or discussed in relation to the development of care services (Allan, 2000; Bamford and Bruce, 2000; Reid, Ryan and Enderby, 2001; Killick and Allan, 2001; Nolan *et al.*, 2002), the definition of quality of life measurement tools (Bond, 1999; Bond and Corner, 2001), understanding the emotional consequences of dementia (Mills,

1997) and the role 'others' play in assisting the expression of self (Killick, 1994, 1996, 1997; Sabat and Harré 1992; Killick and Allan, 2001; Sabat, 2001).

Things have changed recently in attitudes towards people with dementia in general and to communication in particular. A popular idea, not so long ago, was that when a person with dementia said something that did not make sense to those caring for them, it was the fault of the dementia, and by extension, the fault of the person with the diagnosis (Feil, 1993). However, within a broadening critique of the biomedical model of dementia (Lyman, 1989; Kitwood, 1993) and the development of a philosophy of person-centred care (Kitwood and Bredin, 1992; Kitwood, 1997a) communication 'problems' have been re-located into the realm of interpersonal relationships. This has occurred at a number of levels.

The argument that the process of dementia should be understood as a dialectical interplay between neurological impairment and psychological state (Kitwood, 1989; Kitwood and Bredin, 1992) has shifted attention on to the psychological experience of people with dementia. Although this perspective imagines people with dementia as somewhat passive, they are (unlike previous ideas about dementia) acknowledged to exist within social relationship to others. For people with dementia these 'others' are frequently care workers in health and social care settings, and so further arguments can be made about the need for these workers to improve their communication practices (Kitwood, 1997a). In addition, it has been suggested that psychological interventions might be beneficial to people with dementia, in particular to help them manage the negative impact social context may have on them (Cheston and Bender, 1999).

Secondly, there has been an explicit focus on communication with people with dementia. Many leading care practitioners in the UK believe it is possible to communicate effectively with most people with dementia, most of the time, if we take the trouble to listen (Goldsmith, 1996). This sea-change in debates about communication, from 'them and their problem' to 'us and our practices', has also been seen in the strategies put forward to improve the ways we seek to communicate with people with dementia (Feil, 1993; Killick, 1994). The idea that 'we' (i.e. those without dementia) must ourselves deliberately and consciously adapt in order make communication succeed, to find 'cooperative strategies' (Sabat, 2001, p. 39), supports the idea that taking responsibility for our part in communication with people with dementia may help us to manage an experience we may otherwise feel compelled to turn away from (Kitwood, 1997a; Killick and Allan, 2001). Yet it is worth the effort, for it is at this face-to-face level of interaction that people with dementia may be empowered:

> One of the major ways they [people with dementia] are disadvantaged is through losing control over how interactions and communication arise and unfold (Killick and Allan, 2001, p. 54).

A specific interaction in which people with dementia might be said to be disadvantaged has been the focus of a third area of debate. Interpersonal relationships have been introduced into discussions about how 'awareness' is determined amongst people with dementia. This is evident in the criticism levelled at standardized tests that are used in clinical settings to determine the levels of awareness possessed by people with dementia. It is argued that such tests are limited to investigation of the impact of dementia on certain functions, rather than on how dementia 'affects persons living in the world' (Sabat, 2001, p. 10). 'Living in the world' draws attention to social context and the interactions which people with dementia share, the ways others react and how people with dementia respond to these reactions (Sabat, 2002). Specifically, these include interactions people with dementia have with partners and friends, the contact they have with health services and the representations of dementia held within the general socio-cultural milieu (Clare, 2002). Thus it is argued that awareness cannot be explained by individual factors alone but must also include 'the attitudes and behaviour of those around the person with dementia' (Killick and Allan, 2001, p. 269).

The interpersonal domain in general and communication in particular must be borne in mind in discussing any experience of people with dementia, including their experience of pain. Moreover, the assertion that the degree of awareness any person with dementia has may be 'knowledge-based, rather than neurological or psychological in origin' (Clare, 2002, p. 304) directs us to consider our own roles as well as the 'local grammar' (Harré, 1998) of the settings in which people with dementia live and in which they may experience pain.

This is a theme echoed by Goldsmith (1996). He undertook a consultation exercise amongst leading practitioners, researchers and a small number of people with dementia about their views on the possibility of communication. The conclusions of this exercise clearly place the onus for promoting communication on 'us' rather than 'them':

> It is possible to be involved in meaningful communication with the vast majority of people with dementia but we must be able to enter their world, understand their sense of pace and time, recognise the problems of distraction and realise that there are many ways in which people with dementia express themselves, and it is our responsibility to learn how to recognise these (Goldsmith, 1996, p. 165).

This understanding of communication suggests that the subjectivity of people with dementia relies upon communication relationships (see also Killick, 1994, 1996, 1997; Allan, 2000; Killick and Allan, 2001; Sabat, 2001, 2002). The difficulties that may arise in 'us' understanding what is being communicated are not, as in the biomedical model, located solely in explanations of neurological impairment.

The development of ideas in this area has also involved a focus on non-verbal communication. In these discussions, the interpretative work of those seeking to understand the subjectivity of people with dementia is given a high degree of emphasis. Non-verbal communication has been given less attention, and this may reflect the kinds of difficulties that are involved. For example, a study into the pain experienced by people with dementia found that observation of behaviour was the only reliable method (Marzinski, 1991, p. 27). The idea that the behaviour of people with dementia should be viewed as a form of communication is evident in current thinking in this area (Killick and Allan, 2001). An example of this is seen in discussions about 'wandering' (Cayton, 1997, p. 14) where the origin of problems faced by people with dementia are identified not in their dementia but in 'dysfunctional social interactions' (Sabat, 2001, p. 2).

A desire to understand the subjectivity of people with dementia and enhance communication lies behind Kitwood's (1997b, pp. 15–17) suggestion of six 'access routes' by which to do so. These are:

- Accounts written by people with dementia.
- Careful listening to what people say in some kind of interview or group context.
- Attending carefully and imaginatively to what people say and do in the course of their everyday life.
- Consulting those who have undergone an illness with dementia-like features.
- The use of our own poetic imagination.
- The possibility of using role play.

These suggestions are intended to highlight a range of methods that can be used to create a 'collage' of subjective experience and, importantly, involve not only what people with dementia say or do but also what we ourselves observe in ourselves in our reactions to people with dementia and the idea of dementia as an experience.

Research

During 1997 I undertook semi-structured interviews with 14 people with a confirmed diagnosis of dementia who were regularly attending one of 4 day-care settings in central Scotland. Part of my fieldwork strategy was to spend time with the four cohorts of attenders 'doing day care' over a series of weeks before undertaking the interviews. During this 'familiarity phase' my main intention was to develop a rapport with attenders and seek to recruit those who gave (what I judged to be) informed consent to do so (Reid, 1999; Reid, Ryan and Enderby, 2001). Interviews were also conducted with 22 care workers. The substantive focus was to encourage care workers to reveal their personal views about dementia and to describe the ways they learned about people with dementia from the point when they started attending the respective day-care services.

My theoretical commitment and moral conviction was to encourage attenders to describe themselves in ways of their own choosing. I did not want to impose a dementia label on the people that I met. With this in mind I decided that I would not use the words 'dementia' or 'Alzheimer's disease' with attenders unless they introduced these terms themselves. My interview schedule was thus structured so as to encourage attenders to talk about themselves 'in the past', 'in the present' and 'in the future' – if possible, in equal measure during the interviews. However, it was only when I reflected on my field notes that I realized care workers in the setting were unwittingly engaged in a 'conspiracy' which had the effect of denying attenders their experiences of dementia.

I shall draw upon two strands of data. Firstly, I highlight some of the ways in which care workers embargoed use of the term 'dementia' and its synonyms. Secondly, I highlight how day-care attenders spoke about themselves as 'older' people.

Care workers and mentioning dementia

Care workers were asked whether or not they used the word 'dementia' in any of their conversations with attenders. None of the care workers had ever discussed this particular issue with colleagues, but there was a consensus amongst them that the word dementia should not be used with attenders unless there were good reasons. For example, Julie and Marjorie knew that Ernest had been told by his GP that he had a diagnosis of Alzheimer's disease. As he knew this and spoke openly about it, Julie and Marjorie felt they could legitimately speak with Ernest about his dementia. Marjorie had further experience of another man who had spoken about his dementia. Her opinion was that it was okay to talk with attenders like this about their dementia as they were 'early onset people who are still aware of their situation'.

Beatrice said that she had also once talked with an attender about his diagnosis. She had done this when 'reality orientation' had been an influential philosophy in dementia care and had not done it again since. Her opinion was that using the word should be based upon a 'judgement . . . of whose needs you're meeting' although she admitted not knowing whether this was 'the right or the wrong approach'.

In general these care workers were extremely cautious about using the term 'dementia' with day-care attenders, and had done so only when it had been mentioned first. Sandy did not think she had ever used the word with attenders. She explained that the primary reason for not doing so was because of uncertainty about what an attender's reaction might be:

> It depends on the person themselves. Some of them can accept, they know that there is something wrong and then of course there's others then that live in their own wee world and just do think that it's everything else that's wrong about them and it's no' them. So there are some I suppose that you could try and explain to but then there's them who just wouldnae accept it. So you've really got to be careful who you're saying to. (Sandy: 2)

These care workers raised two important issues that seem to have framed their decisions about using the term 'dementia'. The first is about their knowledge of attenders' own acknowledgement of their diagnoses. The second is about the likely reaction of attenders to the word itself.

Julie said that as care workers they did not know what GPs had said to attenders, not what the respective families had told them. Joanna said that she did not want to be the one to mention dementia for the first time to an attender. She also felt that it might be possible to discover what an attender had been told by contacting the relevant social worker. However, no care workers said they had actively sought to discover an attender's knowledge of their diagnosis in this way.

There was a concern amongst care workers about the impact that speaking about dementia might have on attender who was not aware of his or her diagnosis. The belief that 'it's not for us to tell them' (Debbie: 10) was a conclusion that some care workers appeared to have reached after having first considered what the 'impact' might be.

> How do we know, how do you know that this person hasn't been told? How do you know? And even if you do, even if they have been told, if they're not retaining it then they'll be hearing this for the first time. That must be horrendous. (Andrea)

What care workers did feel responsible for, in this context, was managing the fears that attenders might have, regardless of whether attenders had made a link between their fears and their diagnosis of dementia. This was demonstrated in their shared concern to avoid responsibility for magnifying any fears a person might have by mentioning dementia. Care workers gave a number of such reasons for not speaking about dementia with day-care attenders. The following excerpt indicates the kind of concerns that Miriam and Sandy shared about the reaction of attenders to hearing the word:

> M: Never to the person . . . because dementia, it's – these are people of a generation that when you talk about mental illness.
>
> S: You're talkin' about the loony-bin!
>
> M: You're talkin' about the loony-bin. You're talkin' about the poor's house. They're locked away, they cannae be out in the community . . . But to use the word 'dementia'? No, it would be demeaning, I think. It would be throwin' mental illness in these people's faces and they couldnae take it. (Miriam and Sandy)

Andrea had the same concern, that attenders might feel 'hopeless' if they were told that dementia was responsible for their experiences of, for example, memory loss. Joanna's reason was that attenders might ask further questions that would be difficult to answer, or that they might deny it. Both possibilities were uncomfortable prospects. Maggie had never heard an attender use the word, and she was as circumspect as her colleagues about using the word directly with attenders. This was a judgement that originated more in 'a feeling' than because of specific reasons:

> I mean you never ever get a client saying 'I've got dementia'. You never ever get that . . . If somebody came in and I heard them saying to a resident or to a client in day care 'Oh, I mean, do you not realize you've got dementia?' I mean I would actually take them aside and say 'Look! You're not really supposed to say that'. (Maggie)

Thus care workers said they did not use the word dementia to explain to attenders why they might be experiencing (what to care workers were clearly) symptoms of dementia. In the excerpt below Marjorie summarizes the position care workers found themselves in and the conclusion many came to:

> I wouldn't dream of mentioning it . . . If they don't have any insight and the family haven't discussed it with them and the GP hasn't discussed it with them I don't think it's my place to – to say they have dementia. (Marjorie)

Explaining memory loss

Care workers agreed that they were often asked by attenders to explain why they experienced memory loss or why they were 'here', in day care. These questions posed a challenge to care workers. For example, Julie said that it was not only the word dementia that had to be avoided:

> We don't use [the word] dementia, we don't talk about the social work department, we don't talk about [the local] hospital, we don't talk about day care . . . Because they don't want to be reminded, the people that we look after, you know, and they don't want to be classed generally as people who suffer dementia. (Julie)

With the absence of dementia or any other words that might be associated with it, care workers had developed a seemingly coherent alternative explanation to offer to attenders who asked questions. Typically this involved suggesting to attenders that their experiences of memory loss were 'normal'. For example, Miriam provided an anecdote of how she and Sandy had responded to Jan, a woman who had previously been an attender at Service A:

> I mean Jan was really bad, her short-term memory, there was nothin' there. And she would say 'Oh lassies! what's wrong wi' me? What's gone wrong wi' me?' And we used to sit and be quite candid wi' her, hey. We'll say 'Well Jan, you're ninety-two. And these things can happen but when you're young, you've got a lot of brain cells and you're sharp' I said, 'but when you get, especially – you're into overtime, ken! You're into injury time, well into injury time. You're only allowed threescore years and ten. You ken your bible!' I says 'God' You're ninety two!' 'Oh I never feel ninety-two.' I says 'No, you think you're sixteen, Jan, we ken that. But it's part of the ageing process and these cells all die'. I mean we're explainin' dementia to her without mentionin' the word. We're actually tellin' her she's got this deteriorating illness and it's no' an illness, it's age . . . It's comin' wi' old age and what can she expect? And that she's not to be worried about it because we're here for her. 'I don't know what I'd do without you lassies. I could tell you anything'. Ken, and this is the relationship you build. The fear's still there, of course it is. I mean it's a terrible thing. But it takes the edge off their fear for them. (Miriam and Sandy)

This link between memory loss and the normal process of ageing was a strategy that all care workers said they had employed at one time or another. For example, Sheila explained the approach she used:

> I would say to somebody 'This is because you are getting older. These things happen, don't worry about it. We can maybe try one or two ways to keep your memory going.' And I would work that way. (Sheila)

This explanation appeared to be one that made sense to attenders:

> If a client was in there [day care] and turned around and I said to them 'How are you doing? I saw you last time you were in' and she said, 'I can't remember!' I'd say, maybe just 'A bad day – your memory's not as good as it was' . . . I mean they know, as they get older their memory's not as good. (Maggie)

Bonnie also drew attention to the understanding that attenders had come to themselves about their experiences of memory loss:

> And there isnae even any point in saying because it would be 'What's dementia?' or 'What's this? I'm just forgettin'!' They have this belief in theirselves so I don't see why I should be judge and say 'Oh you have dementia. It's a criterion and you're in it. You fit in.' Cause it's no' that. I think it's what everybody wants to believe. And if their belief is 'Oh I'm forgettin'! I'm gettin' old', I say 'Oh well. It comes to us all sometime.' And that's the way I get round it. (Bonnie)

This approach to respecting the account of memory loss that attenders had developed was endorsed by Julie, Marjorie and Miriam. In their cases it was particularly important for attenders at their services to have understandings of memory loss that were compatible with the prevailing ethos that attenders ought to feel like 'guests' or 'visitors' in these settings:

> They're our friends and they come to visit and that's how we like to keep it. We don't like people to think that we are solely here just to look after them. We want their friendship, we want a rapport to be built up between us so you can't say, you know, you're coming to day care because you've got dementia and I'm here to look after you. (Julie)

Although linking memory loss with age was the primary way in which care workers responded to attenders' concerns, some care workers were keen to give as 'honest' an account as possible. In the excerpt below Andrea describes her strategy:

> I think if I'm honest I would rather not say it [the word dementia] because I think that people just look at it and they think there's no' going to be any way out of this. There's no' going to be a tablet, they're no' going to get better. This is going to get worse. So I do try – maybe I'm copping out, I don't know, 'When you get this wee bit older your memory does go. If you're worrying about things then things'll be that wee bit more harder to concentrate on and . . .' But if they say to me 'Will I get better?' or if they say – a lot of people say to

me 'Will I get worse?' or 'Am I going to be like her one day?' I can always just answer as truthfully as I can and just say 'No two people are the same. There is nothing to say that you will be like that.' (Andrea)

Conclusion

The belief, expressed some years ago, that people with dementia 'have much to teach us' (Cohen and Eisdorfer, 1986, p. 22) has been elegantly vindicated with the publication of academic articles by people with dementia (Friedell and Bryden, 2002; Sterin, 2002). Furthermore, advocacy services for people with dementia now exist (e.g. Westminster Advocacy Service for Senior Residents (see Jones, 2004)) and a self-advocacy organization (*www.dasninternational.org*) has recently emerged. Also, the UK Alzheimer's Society now has people with dementia at the heart of its internal policy-making.

However, what I have tried to show in this chapter is that for some people with dementia, what they know about themselves can be controlled by other people. Communication can be difficult and it can involve discussion of emotional subjects, such as a person's dementia and what this means to them. Yet, if health-care professionals consider their own role in this communication and think about how they might adapt their own practices to ensure that a person's experience is heard and valued, then it is more likely than not that a person with dementia who experiences pain will have this recognized. As the examples of the attitudes of care workers in this chapter show, however a person's experience is framed, it is most important that that person is heard.

Summary

- **Assessment:** Nurses should focus on their own assumptions, fears and thoughts about dementia as well as adapting to try and understand whether a person with dementia is experiencing pain.
- **Planning:** Nurses should consider all forms of communication – verbal, non-verbal (including behaviour) and their own observations – as valid sources of information about whether or not a person with dementia is experiencing pain.
- **Implementation:** People with dementia vary in their communicative abilities depending on the impairment caused by their condition, the impact this has on nurses' ability and willingness to try to understand what is being communicated, and the possible effects of pain being experienced. Creative

methods may be needed to record and act upon this accumulated knowledge.

- **Evaluation:** A genuine and ongoing attention to individuals and what they are communicating will provide an essential stream of information about whether or not a person is experiencing pain.

References

Allan, K. (2000) *Communication and Consultation: Exploring Ways for Staff to Involve People with Dementia in Developing Services.* Joseph Rowntree Foundation and the Policy Press, Bristol.

Bamford, L. and Bruce, E. (2000) Defining the outcomes of community care: the perspectives of older people with dementia and their carers. *Ageing and Society,* **20**(5), 543–70.

Bender, M.P. and Cheston, R. (1997) Inhabitants of a lost kingdom: a model of the subjective experiences of dementia. *Ageing and Society,* **17**, 513–32.

Binstock, R.H. (ed.) (1992) *Dementia and Aging: Ethics, Values and Policy Choices.* Johns Hopkins University Press, Baltimore.

Bond, J. (1999) Quality of life for people with dementia: approaches to the challenge of measurement. *Ageing and Society,* **19**, 561–79.

Bond, J. and Corner, L. (2001) Researching dementia: are there unique methodological challenges for health services research? *Ageing and Society,* **21**, 95–116.

Cayton, H. (1997) Hunting in the dark. *Journal of Dementia Care,* **5**(6), 14–15.

Cheston, R. and Bender, M. (1999) *Understanding Dementia: The Man with the Worried Eyes.* Jessica Kingsley, London.

Clare, L. (2002) Developing awareness about awareness in early-stage dementia: the role of psychosocial factors. *Dementia. International Journal of Social Research and Practice,* **1**(3), 295–312.

Cohen, D. and Eisdorfer, C. (1986) *The Loss of Self. A Family Resource for the Care of Alzheimer's Disease and Related Disorders.* W.W. Norton, New York.

Feil, N. (1993) *The Validation Breakthrough: Simple Techniques for Communicating with People with Alzheimer's-Type Dementia.* Health Professions Press, Baltimore.

Friedell, M. and Bryden (Boden), C. (2002) A word from two turtles. *Dementia. International Journal of Social Research and Practice,* **1**(2), 131–3.

Goldsmith, M. (1996) *Hearing the Voice of People with Dementia. Opportunities and Obstacles.* Jessica Kingsley, Bristol.

Harré, R. (1998) *The Singular Self: An Introduction to the Psychology of Personhood.* Sage, Thousand Oaks, CA.

Hofman, A., Rocca, W.A., Brayne, C., Breteler, M.M.B., Clarke, M., Cooper, B., Copeland, J.R.M., Dartigues, J.F., Da Silva Droux, A., Hagnell, O., H/Meeren, T.J.,

Engedal, K., Jonker, C., Lindesay, J., Lobo, A., Mann, A.H., Molsa, P.K., Morgan, K., O'Connor, D.W., Sulkava, R., Kay, D.W.K. and Amaducci, L. (1991) The prevalence of dementia in Europe: a collaborative study of 1980–1990 findings. *International Journal of Epidemiology*, **20**(3), 736–48.

Jones, J. (2004) *Adding Value Through Advocacy. Report of an Investigation to Find the Benefits WASSR Brings to the Community and to Statutory Service Providers in Westminster.* Westminster Advocacy Service for Senior Residents.

Killick, J. (1994) *Please Five Me Back My Personality: Writing and Dementia.* Dementia Services Development Centre, University of Stirling.

Killick, J. (1997) Communication: a matter of life and death of the mind. *Journal of Dementia Care*, **5**(5), 14–16.

Killick, J. and Allan, K. (2001) *Communication and the Care of People with Dementia.* Open University Press, Buckingham.

Kitwood, T. (1989) Brain, mind and dementia: with particular reference to Alzheimer's. *Disease. Ageing and Society*, **9**, 1–15.

Kitwood, T. (1993) *Towards the reconstruction of an organic mental disorder*, in *Worlds of Illness*, Ch. 8 (ed. A. Radley), pp. 143–60. Routledge, London.

Kitwood, T. (1997a) *Dementia Reconsidered: The Person Comes First.* Open University Press, Buckingham.

Kitwood, T. (1997b) The experience of dementia. *Aging and Mental Health*, **1**(1), 13–22.

Kitwood, T. and Bredin, K. (1992) Towards a theory of dementia care: personhood and well-being. *Ageing and Society*, **12**, 269–87.

Lyman, K. (1989) Bringing the social back in. A critique of the biomedicalization of dementia. *The Gerontologist*, **29**(5), 597–605.

Marzinski, L.R. (1991) The tragedy of dementia: clinically assessing pain in the confused, nonverbal elderly. *Journal of Gerontological Nursing*, **17**(6), 25–8.

Mills, M. (1997) Narrative identity and dementia: a study of emotion and narrative in older people with dementia. *Ageing and Society*, **17**(6), 673–98.

Nolan, M., Ryan, T., Enderby, P. and Reid, D. (2002) Towards a more inclusive vision of dementia care practice and research. *Dementia. The International Journal of Social Research and Practice*, **1**(2), 193–212.

Reid, D. (1999) *Conscience and consent: involving people with dementia in social research.* Oral paper presentation, Society for the Study of Social Problems annual meeting, Chicago, IL. August 1999.

Reid, D., Ryan, T. and Enderby, P. (2001) What does it mean to listen to people with dementia? *Disability and Society*, **16**(3), 377–92.

Rosengren, K.E. (2000) *Communication. An Introduction.* Sage, London.

Sabat, S.R. (2001) *The Experience of Alzheimer's Disease.* Blackwell, Oxford.

Sabat, S.R. (2002) Epistemological issues in the study of insight in people with Alzheimer's disease. *Dementia. The International Journal of Social Research and Practice*, **I**(3), 279–94.

Sabat, S.R. and Harré, R. (1992) The construction and deconstruction of self in Alzheimer's disease. *Ageing and Society*, **12**, 443–61.

Sterin, G.J. (2002) Essay on a word. A lived experience of Alzheimer's disease. *Dementia. The International Journal of Social Research and Practice*, **1**(1), 7–10.

Woods, R. (2001) Discovering the person with Alzheimer's disease: cognitive, emotional and behavioural aspects. *Aging and Mental Health*, **5**(Suppl 1): s7–16.

Web sites

Alzheimer's Disease International: <*http://www.alz.co.uk/*>

Alzheimer's Society (UK): <*http://www.alzheimers.org.uk/*>

Dementia Advocacy and Support Network International: <*http://www. dasninternational.org*>

Acute on chronic pain

6

Margaret Dunham

Introduction

Acute pain is a symptom of nociceptive damage; something injured needs repair, and when it is repaired the pain goes away. For many older adults, however, the reality is that chronic pain is a part of daily existence, with acute flare-ups a daily fear. Chronic pain is commonly associated with many age-related conditions, with rheumatoid arthritis top of the list. The incidence of Parkinson's disease, stroke and many other neurological disorders increases with age. Diabetes and cancer are also likely to contribute to the decline of many older people.

It is the norm is that many older people suffer with chronic pain on a daily basis; epidemiological studies support this (Helme and Gibson, 1999; Kung, Gibson and Helme, 1999; Cramer *et al.*, 2000; Landi *et al.*, 2001; Chodosh *et al.*, 2004; Won *et al.*, 2004; Breivik *et al.*, 2006). Consequently many people believe that pain is a normal part of growing old, and older people are largely excluded from pharmacological study of new analgesics (Closs *et al.*, 2004).

Our elders are important to society, and it should be a fundamental right for everyone, regardless of age or infirmity, to have access to adequate pain relief. Pain of any kind may be a contributory factor in reducing quality of life and there may be consequent reduction in independence for older people, so keeping our elders relatively pain-free is bound to be beneficial both for them and for society. Older people themselves may be reluctant to approach heath-care professionals because of becoming 'bothersome' (Yong *et al.*, 2001). The issue here is that though existing chronic pain may be lived with, and barely coped with, acute pain on top of this can ensure that all potential coping strategies are exhausted.

However, little research is available to support older peoples' pain management, particularly of acute on chronic pain.

What is pain?

In order to embrace the phenomenon of acute on chronic pain, it is important to revisit the definitions widely used in pain management. For the lay person pain may have a different meaning as a term in common usage, so although they are not exhaustive these definitions may help in establishing a plan of care and mutual goals.

When McCaffrey (1979) defined acute pain, little did she envisage the effect it would have on nursing care all over the world (Table 6.1). This must be the best-known nursing mantra of all and, although it was initially intended for cancer pain sufferers, it holds true for pain of all genres. Before this health-care professionals had seen themselves as the primary authority on what is essentially a subjective and personal experience. Practical limitations of this definition may be flawed for many client groups, particularly those unable to express themselves in the same language as their carers. Older people, people with cognitive impairment and the very young also rely on the carer's opinion of their subjective pain experience. Nurses have been noted as consistently underscoring their patients' pain experience as compared with their patients self-report (Bergh and Sjostrom, 1999; Bennet *et al.*, 2006). However, the sentiment of centring the focus of pain assessment on the patient's own account remains fundamental to the implementation of good pain relief.

Table 6.1 Definitions of pain

General definition	Pain is an unpleasant sensory associated with actual or potential tissue damage and defined in terms of that damage	Merskey and Bogduk (1994)
Acute pain	Pain is what the experiencing person says it is and it occurs whenever the experiencing patient says it does	McCaffrey (1979)
Chronic pain	That which persists beyond the expected healing time, serves no useful purpose and has no identifiable physical cause	Merskey and Bogduk (1994)

Chronic pain is often described as a disease in its own right, whereas acute pain is the symptom. For an older person the increasing incidence of disease and likelihood of surgical procedures add up to the potential for debilitating chronic pain. Accumulating evidence links the increased frequency of chronic pain as a direct consequence of surgical events (Perkins and Kehlet, 2000; Kehlet, Jensen and Woolf, 2006). Osteoarthritis and rheumatoid arthritis are the most common cause of chronic pain, and are more frequent with increasing age (Breivik et al., 2006). In most individuals the experience of chronic pain does not preclude the occurrence of acute pain episodes, which may or may not be directly associated with the cause of the chronic pain. The issue of distinguishing acute from chronic pain inevitably becomes more complicated with the co-morbidity and polypharmacy of ageing. There is recent evidence that for older people the usual distinction between acute (nociceptive) and chronic (neuropathic) pain may not be as clear as once thought, particularly when considered from the patient's perspective of neuropathic symptoms and the clinician's observation of the diagnosis (Rasmussen et al., 2004; Bennet et al., 2006). This may also reflect the perception of older people in pain where such a clear distinction is difficult.

Much is written about the importance of managing acute pain; similarly, there is a plethora of advice on cancer pain (Drayer, Henderson and Reidenberg, 1999). Acute pain for cancer patients is known as **breakthrough pain**, but unfortunately there is no such clear definition for chronic pain sufferers. The terms **breakthrough**, **incidental**, **transient** and **episodic** are all commonly used in the literature. The European Association of Palliative Care (EAPC) prefers the term **episodic pain**, which, though possibly ambiguous, forms part of a strategy that may have transferable and suitable aspects for managing acute on chronic pain (Mercadante et al., 2002).

Assessing acute on chronic pain

Assessing pain is a skilled and complex procedure. For the registered nurse it carries with it the weight of responsibility to ensure adequate appropriate treatment for the client via direct management strategies and through collaboration with the multi-disciplinary team (Frampton, 2003). Older people's pain is complicated, with a potential plethora of disease processes such as rheumatoid disorders and neurological problems often associated with neuropathic pain, the pain caused by damage to the pain pathways (Breivik et al., 2006). The British Pain Society cites examples of chronic conditions which may predispose to episodic acute pain, such as sickle cell disease, haemophilia, refractory angina, osteoporosis, rheumatoid arthritis, vascular disease and pancreatic pain (Collins and Simpson, 2005). Pain syndromes are also increasingly common with age (Lynch, 2000). Cognitive impairment,

Table 6.2 Assessing breakthrough pain

- Do you have any episodes of severe pain?
- How often do they occur? Daily, weekly?
- How long do they last?
- How does it affect you?
- Does it limit your activities at all? Describe.
- Do you avoid anything which you feel may cause this severe pain?
- What helps you, if anything, to take the pain away?

---

though not automatic with age, is more prevalent in this population and this may lead to issues with use of existing pain assessment strategies.

Thus pain may be ubiquitous in the ageing population but remains unique and individual to the person concerned. Each aspect of the pain phenomenon has a meaning and interpretation for their daily living and circumstances. In the absence of a standard definition of a subjective experience, the nurse is reliant on patient report or carer observation. This is further complicated because distinction has to be made between the acute pain and chronic pain experience, the former being one-dimensional and linear, the latter multidimensional and complex.

The suitability of pain assessment tools for acute pain is questioned by clinicians who consider patients may not be able to conceptualize the 0–10 of the visual analogue scale (Gibson, 2006). Use of the words 'mild, moderate, severe' as part of a combined verbal and numerical rating assessment tool is preferred by practitioners in pain management. Both of these may be suitable for the patient solely experiencing acute pain. For the person with more than one type of pain and more than one site of pain, use of combined tools and body diagram, combined with a simple questionnaire (Table 6.2) may be helpful (Fink, 2000).

Learning point

Consider what pain means to you. Make a note of all the adjectives you have used, and heard used, to describe pain.

Case study

Mary is an 82 year old widow who lives independently in her own house. She has osteoporosis and has lost 7 cm in height in the last 10 years. She also suffers with arthritic changes in her hips and knees but is considered unsuitable for surgery because of her pre-existing hypertension and diabetes. She currently takes codeine in the form of co-codamol (codeine 5 mg/paracetamol 500 mg) tablets, 2–4 times daily, but does not find them effective. She does not tolerate ibuprofen or other NSAIDs because of their gastric effects.

Learning point

What are Mary's options for pain management?

The use of multidimensional tools to combine assessing the pain and its life-modifying effects is the preferred option for this client group. Simply asking 'do you have pain?' is unlikely to get a qualified and informative response; the term 'pain' may have other associations, or simply not enter the normal vocabulary of the individual because of a level of stoicism.

In the case study above, Mary's different pain experiences may have their own problems in terms of functional, psychological and emotional effects. The gnawing continuous pain of the degenerating spinal column as described by Mary may be exacerbated by different stimuli from the knee and hip pain which is triggered by walking on uneven surfaces and when climbing steps. Recent comparison of patients with neuropathic and non-neuropathic pain showed surprising similarity in verbal descriptors with 'burning', 'shooting' and 'pricking' common to both groups (Rasmussen et al., 2004). The McGill Pain Assessment tool (described in Chapter 4), which utilizes verbal descriptors, may be appropriate in this instance to give an initial picture of the pain. An understanding of the triggers and precipitating factors in acute pain episodes may be acquired through introduction of a pain diary (Melzack, 1983). Individuals like Mary in the case study may have complicated medical and life histories and it can take skill, time and patience for an experienced pain practitioner to give colour and context to the current situation. Empathy is the key here, seeing the patient as a person by showing genuine interest in the individual as a whole.

Learning point

- Look at the pain assessment tools available in your clinical area. How can they be used for older people with acute on chronic pain? Discuss with your colleagues and members of the multidisciplinary pain team.
- Consider the communication strategies in your clinical area – verbal, written, etc. Are written communications available in alternative forms, such as Braille, large print or audiotape?

Pharmacological treatment options

The WHO analgesic ladder (Figure 6.1) is usually ascended for chronic pain starting with simple analgesics, opioids being the last option; for acute pain the reverse is usually justifiable (WHO, 1996). Some of the newer opioids – methadone, fentanyl, tramadol and others – are beginning to be recognized as useful analgesics for older people, with codeine largely avoided due to the potential for constipation (Dellemijn, van Duijn and vanneste, 1998; Kalso *et al.*, 2003; Fredheim *et al.*, 2006). The general strategy in acute pain is to start with strong opioids and work down the ladder. The required size of 'breakthrough' or 'rescue' dose of opioid for a person with pre-existing chronic pain may seem extravagant, if not dangerous, to the inexperienced health-care professional. An inappropriately small dose of opioid, or even its omission, may lead to pain being poorly managed. Compound this with an acute pain episode and the potential for 'opiophobia' from members of the health-care team; then the situation is likely to prove unsatisfactory.

In our example, Mary is not finding codeine in combination with paracetamol (co-codamol) at all suitable for her needs, but in this situation should she be given different or stronger opioids? What are the alternatives? What can she take for rescue if she walks back home from the shops when the bus fails to turn up and her back hurts, or if she decides to clean all her windows because it is a lovely day

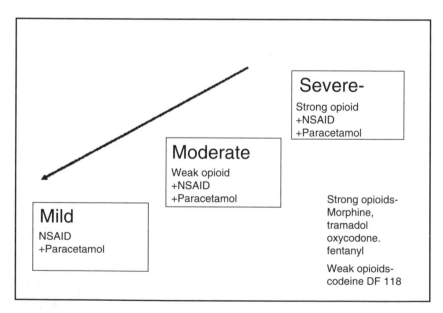

Figure 6.1 The WHO pain control ladder. Treatment starts at the bottom for chronic pain, but at the top for acute pain

and the sun is shining but then overstretches herself? These are the kind of issues which need to be addressed and clearly the multidimensional factors influencing the whole pain experience need to be addressed at a pragmatic level. The British Pain Society recommends that opioids be used as part of an overall strategy for the management of acute on chronic pain with prompt referral to an appropriate specialist (Collins and Simpson, 2005).

Case study

Maureen, aged 69, is a grandmother and part-time carer for her four small grand-children. She has had breast cancer and associated treatment, and takes 150 mg morphine slow-release tablets twice a day for the consequent breast pain. She is admitted to hospital with back pain and is very uncomfortable. What are her options?

Maureen is likely to need much more analgesia for her acute back pain than an opioid-naive person. It is therefore reasonable that her analgesia should be titrated to find a satisfactory level for her. The term **multimodal**, though often applied to the acute pain experience, seems eminently appropriate here since the combination of pharmacological and non-pharmacological strategies may enhance the whole pain and quality of life experience for Maureen (Maier *et al.*, 2002; Kehlet, 1997).

Non-pharmacological treatment options

For the chronic pain sufferer, breakthrough pain after activity or exercise is likely to be inadequately controlled by existing pain medication. Management of acute on chronic pain needs to reflect the individuality of the pain experience; however, the range of usual non-pharmacological treatment options should be considered as part of any primary intervention. For musculoskeletal pain, these non-pharmacological interventions for acute pain may include the usual regimen of rest, elevation, cautious and considered use of heat/cold, followed by supervised gentle exercise and regaining of strength. Supported rehabilitation may prevent development of further chronic pain, loss of productivity or reduced quality of life. In our example Maureen may also need to seek the support of family members if future episodes are to be prevented. Many older people are carers either of older relatives or of grandchildren, and the holistic assessment and management must include this consideration.

The acute pain experience described by chronic pain sufferers, using terms such as 'shooting' or 'stabbing', may be in addition to the underlying pain, forming layers of pain experiences. This is often described as **neuropathic pain** (Jensen *et al.*, 2001; Rasmussen *et al.*, 2004). Neuropathic pain may also be stimulus-dependent, from relatively innocuous stimuli such as heat or cold, referred to as **allodynia** (non-painful stimuli producing pain) or **hyperalgesia** (exaggerated pain response) and can be compared to the breakthrough pain of cancer patients (Svendsen *et al.*, 2005). However, for chronic pain, unlike cancer pain, there should not be a 'monotherapy' of opioids but a structured rehabilitation and education programme of therapies which incorporate alternatives for breakthrough pain and patient preference for what works for them. Pain management education/training may involve education in relaxation, exercise, thought modification and setting of goals (Ersek *et al.*, 2004).

Diagnosis and continuing care

Even with good pain assessment strategies, diagnosis of a painful condition does not guarantee continuing care. In a study of some 372 community-dwelling older adults the population incidence of painful episodes was 33%. The diagnosis of a painful condition did not guarantee continuing care, as only 66% received clinical follow-up (Chodosh *et al.*, 2004). Comparison of older people with and without Alzheimer's disease has shown that acute pain in patients with existing chronic pain conditions appears to be similar for both groups; however, the chronic pain experience for the Alzheimer's group was not as easy to identify (Pickering, Jourdan and Dubray, 2006). It is also postulated that in Alzheimer's disease the NMDA (N-methyl-D-aspartate) receptors may be impaired, thus reducing the potential for central sensitization and unfortunately the potential use of some co-analgesics. In addition, older people may be unable to tolerate some of the simple analgesics, such as NSAIDs, thus limiting options even further (Gibson, 2006). In the absence of a range of pharmacological strategies effective for chronic pain in older people, the use of other strategies such as CBT (cognitive behavioural therapy) and education cannot be ignored. The British Pain Society's provisional recommendations for pain management programmes include strategies for self-management of pain in the community (Williams, 2006).

For a chronic pain sufferer undergoing surgery any existing regime must be acknowledged and the dose, route and so on must be considered, with accommodation in the perioperative period. This may mean switching opioids as part of the preparation for planned surgery, which needs the informed consent and active cooperation of both the patient and the multidisciplinary team. Older people need to be given the same options as their younger counterparts. In a study of postoperative pain management in 224 young and older patients it was found that pain scores and visual analogue scores were not significantly different (Aubrun *et al.*, 2003). In addition, their morphine consumption did not differ significantly.

It is generally acknowledged that patients on surgical wards fare better than those on the medical wards, and older people fare better on surgical wards than medical ones, largely because the nurses on surgical wards are better prepared for managing acute pain. Even on surgical wards the myth of unsuitability of strong opioids can be a barrier to good pain relief (Closs, 1996). Older people, when assessed for cognitive ability and when adequately prepared, are capable of managing their pain effectively with a patient-controlled analgesia delivery system (PCA) (Gagliese *et al.*, 2000). Epidurals are becoming increasingly popular, particularly for lower limb orthopaedic surgery, and when they are effective they provide the best analgesia and the potential for the associated benefits of speedy recovery. If confusion is to be avoided, then for suitable operations the use of an epidural may be the most appropriate option for older people. Continuing this with PCA has proved more than adequate for effective pain management for older people undergoing abdominal surgery (Mann *et al.*, 2000)

Learning point

- Talk to older people in your care. How do they make the distinction between acute and chronic pain?

Opiophobia and other barriers

If opioids remain a useful option then the fear of opioid use needs to be addressed. The global position described by the World Health Organization (1996) is dire, with an estimated four fifths of people with cancer pain dying in unrelieved pain. With cancer pain so poorly recognized, what hope is there for chronic pain? Older people may be denied opioids because of fears of accumulation and CNS depression (AGS Panel on Chronic Pain in Older Persons, 1998).

Lack of knowledge and education has been cited as one of the major barriers to effective pain relief. Nurses historically have had little information in their nurse training to support their understanding of the management of pain (McCaffrey and Ferrell, 1992). Watt-Watson *et al.* (2001) compared nurses' assessment of patients' pain with the self-report of the patients, and found that nurses consistently underscored the patients. Patients in this study with moderate to severe pain received only 47% of the available prescribed analgesia. It is also noted that physicians receive minimal education in managing pain (Green *et al.*, 2002).

The use of a framework or guidelines in this area is therefore appropriate, particularly when knowledge is limited. These must acknowledge the heterogeneity of the ageing population and the varied need for opioid treatment based on individual assessment (Kalso *et al.*, 2003). Unfortunately, sparse and ambiguous data on the long-term benefits of opioid use in chronic non-malignant pain does little to enhance its profile. In a recent retrospective study of 160 patients who had attended a multidisciplinary chronic pain clinic in Denmark 10 years before, little escalation of opioid dose was noted but quality of life and associated depression scores were significantly poorer (Jensen, Thomsen and Hojsted, 2006).

Beyond the humanitarian aspect, one consequence of not acknowledging the limitations these barriers constitute for effective pain management is the potential for litigation. A recent published case from the United States highlights the folly of not acknowledging the issues of pain in the acute hospital, nursing home and community settings (Tucker, 2004). The health-care workers' ignorance and lack of knowledge for prescribing in elder care was not defensible, and the Medical Board of California has ordered its physicians and health-care workers to devote sufficient time to education in pain management.

Learning point

- Consider how you can ensure that older people in your clinical area are enabled to engage with their plan of care.

Conclusion

An essential element of any pain management programme must be education about the potential consequences, including episodes of acute pain. Ensuring patients are active participants in any treatment plan is not just important for compliance but also helps to support and promote healthy living and lifestyle options. The resulting concordance with any treatment programme should lead to improved confidence and enhanced health outcomes. Informed individuals need to know what therapy can do for them, what the positive outcomes may be and the knowledge of any potential deleterious effects. Hypothetically, education leading to acceptance may stimulate increased activity and healthy functioning for the older adult.

Education programmes for clients may include the following (Department of Health, 2001):

- behaviours
- motivation
- belief systems – honesty, tackling fears

- locus of control – teaching skills, accessing resources, use of negotiation
- support networks – family members, expert patient group.

A combination of observation, assessment and reflection, through personal diaries, may inform how the pain behaviour and lifestyle changes affect the older persons' pain experience. If individuals can learn how their pain is modified by drugs and activity, with the aid of members of the multidisciplinary team, then opportunity may be created to work towards mutually agreed and successful outcomes. In the UK the expansion of the 'Expert Patient' programme is an invaluable strategy for self-management and empowerment (Department of Health, 2001).

Without the knowledge and understanding of their own chronic pain regime, individuals will not have the ability to cope with the acute pain experience. The rising age of the population and its increasing potential for dependence on a diminishing younger workforce means that pain should be addressed promptly and not trivialized, in order to maintain dignity and independence. Acknowledging the reality that pain is not an inevitable consequence of ageing, age should not be a barrier to believing the patient's pain account. Older people should be afforded the same credibility and resources as their younger counterparts.

References

AGS Panel on Chronic Pain in Older Persons (1998) The management of chronic pain in older persons. *Journal of the American Geriatrics Society*, **46**, 635–51.

Aubrun, F., Bunge, D., Langeron, O., Saillant, G., Coriat, P. and Riou, B. (2003) Post-operative morphine consumption in the elderly patient. *Anesthesiology*, **99**(1), 160–5.

Bennett, M.I., Smith, B.H., Torrance, N. and Lee, A.J. (2006) Can pain be more or less neuropathic? Comparison of symptom assessment tools with ratings of certainty by clinicians. *Pain*, **122**, 289–94.

Bergh, I. and Sjostrom, B. (1999) A comparative study of nurses' and elderly patients' ratings of pain and pain tolerance. *Journal of Gerontological Nursing*, **25**, 30–6.

Breivik, H., Collett, B., Ventafridda, V., Cohen, R. and Gallacher, D. (2006) Survey of chronic pain in Europe: prevalence, impact on daily life and treatment. *European Journal of Pain*, **10**, 287–333.

Chodosh, J., Solomon, D.H., Roth, C.P., Chang, J.T., MacLean, C.H., Ferrell, B.A., Shekelle, P.G. and Wenger, N.S. (2004) The quality of medical care provided to vulnerable older patients with chronic pain. *Journal of the American Geriatrics Society*, **52**(5), 756–61.

Closs, S.J. (1996) Pain and elderly patients: a survey of nurses' knowledge and experiences. *Journal of Advanced Nursing*, **23**(2), 237–42.

Closs, S.J., Barr, B., Briggs, M., Cash, K. and Seers, K. (2004) A comparison of five pain assessment scales for nursing home residents with varying degrees of cognitive impairment. *Journal of Pain and Symptom Management*, **27**(3), 196–204.

Collins, A. and Simpson, K. (2005) *Recommendations for the Appropriate Use of Opioids in Patients with Chronic Non-Cancer Related Pain*. British Pain Society, London. Available at <*http://www.britishpainsociety.org*>, accessed 07.07.2006.

Cramer, G.W., Galer, B., Mendelson, M.A. and Thompson, G.D. (2000) A drug use evaluation of selected opioid and nonopioid analgesics in the nursing facility setting. *Journal of the American Geriatric Society*, **48**(4), 398–404.

Dellemijn, P.L.I., van Duijn, H. and Vanneste, J.A.L. (1998) Prolonged treatment with transdermal fentanyl in neuropathic pain. *Lancet*, **349**, 753–8.

Department of Health (2001) *The Expert Patient: A New Approach to Chronic Disease Management for the 21st Century*. Department of Health, London.

Drayer, R.A., Henderson, J. and Reidenberg, M. (1999) Barriers to better pain control in hospitalized patients. *Journal of Pain and Symptom Management*, **17**(6), 434–40.

Ersek M., Turner J.A., Cain K.C., Kemp C.A. (2004) Chronic pain self-management for older adults: a randomised controlled trial. *BMC Geriatrics*. Available at <*http://www.biomedcentral.com/1471-2318/4/7*>, accessed 03.07.06.

Fink, R. (2000) Pain assessment: the corner stone to optimal pain management. *BUMC Proceedings*, **13**, 236–9.

Frampton, M. (2003) Experience assessment and management of pain in people with dementia. *Age and Ageing*, **32**(3), 248–51.

Fredheim, O.M.S., Kaasa, S., Dale, P., Klepstad, P., Landro, N.I. and Borchgrevink, P.C. (2006) Opioid switching from oral slow release morphine to oral methadone may improve pain control in chronic non-malignant pain: a nine-month follow-up study. *Palliative Medicine*, **20**, 35–41.

Gagliese, L., Jackson, M., Ritvo, P., Wowk, A. and Katz, J. (2000) Age is not an impediment to effective use of patient-controlled analgesia by surgical patients. *Anesthesiology*, **93**(3), 601–10.

Gibson, S.J. (2006) Older people's pain. *Pain, Clinical Updates*, **14**, 3.

Green, C.R., Wheeler, J.R.C., LaPorte, F., Marchant, B. and Guerrero, E. (2002) How well is chronic pain managed? Who does it well? *Pain Medicine*, **3**(1), 56–65.

Helme R.D. and Gibson S.J. (1999) The epidemiology of pain in older people, in *Epidemiology of Pain* (eds I.K. Crombie, P.R. Croft, S.J. Linton, L. LeResche, M. Von Korff), p. 103. IASP Press, Seattle.

Jensen, M.K., Thomsen, A.B. and Hojsted, J. (2006) 10-year follow up of chronic non-malignant pain patients: opioid use, health related quality of life and health care utilization. *European Journal of Pain*, **10**, 423–33.

Jensen, T.S., Gottrup, H., Kasch, H., Nikolajsen, L., Terkelse, A.J. and Witting, N. (2001) Has basic research contributed to chronic pain treatment? *Acta Anaesthesiologica Scandinavica*, **45**, 1128–35.

Kalso, E., Allan, L., Dellemijn, P.L.I., Faura, C.C., Ilias, W.K., Jensen, T.S., Perrot, S., Plaghki, l.H. and Zenz, M. (2003) Recommendations for using opioids in chronic non-cancer pain. *European Journal of Pain*, **7**, 381–6.

Kehlet, H. (1997) Multimodal approach to control postoperative pathophysiology and rehabilitation. *British Journal of Anaesthesia*, **78**, 606–17.

Kehlet, H., Jensen, T.S. and Woolf, C.J. (2006) Persistent post-surgical pain: risk factors and prevention. *The Lancet*, **367**, 1618–25.

Kung, F., Gibson, S.J. and Helme, R.D. (1999) Factors associated with analgesic and psychotropic medications use by community-dwelling older people with chronic pain. *Australian and New Zealand Journal of Public Health*, **23**(5), 471–4.

Landi, F., Onder, G., Cesari, M., Gambassi, G., Steel, K., Russi, A., Lattanzio, F. and Bernabei, R. (2001) Pain management in frail, community-living elderly patients. *Archives of Internal Medicine*, **161**, 2721–4.

Lynch, D. (2000) Geriatric pain, in *Practical Management of Pain*, 3rd edn (ed. P. Raj), Mosby, London.

McCaffrey, M. (1979) *Nursing Management of the Client with Pain*, 2nd edn. Lippincott, Philadelphia.

McCaffrey, M. and Ferrell, B.R. (1992) Opioid analgesics: nurses' knowledge of doses and psychological dependence. *Journal of Nursing Staff Development*, **8**(2), 77–84.

Maier, C., Hildebrandt, J., Klinger, R., Henrich-Eberl, C. and Lindena, G. (2002) Morphine responsiveness, efficacy and tolerability in chronic non-tumor associated pain-results of a double-blind placebo-controlled trial (MONTAS). *Pain*, **97**, 223–33.

Mann, C., Pouzeratte, Y., Boccara, G., Peccoux, C., Vergne, C., Brunat, G., Domergue, J., Millat, B. and Colson, P. (2000) Comparison of intravenous or epidural patient-controlled analgesia in the elderly after major abdominal surgery. *Anesthesiology*, **92**(2), 433–41.

Melzack, R. (1983) *Pain Measurement and Assessment*. Raven Press, New York.

Mercadante, S., Radbruch, L., Caraceni, A., Cherny, N., Kaasa, S., Nauck, F., Ripamonti, C. and De Conno, F. (2002) Steering committee of the European Association for Palliative Care (EAPC) research network. Episodic (breakthrough) pain: consensus conference of an expert working group of the European Association for Palliative Care. *Cancer*, **94**(3), 832–9.

Mersky H. and Bogduk N. (1994) *Classification of Chronic Pain*, 2nd edn. IASP Press, Seattle.

Perkins, F.M. and Kehlet, H. (2000) Chronic pain as an outcome of surgery: a review of predictive factors. *Anesthesiology*, **93**, 1123–33.

Pickering, G., Jourdan, D. and Dubray, C. (2006) Acute versus chronic pain treatment in Alzheimer's disease. *European Journal of Pain*, **10**, 379–84.

Rasmussen, P.V., Sindrup, S.H., Jensen, T.S. and Bach, F.W. (2004) Symptoms and signs in patients with suspected neuropathic pain. *Pain*, **110**, 461–9.

Svendsen, K.B., Andersen, S., Arnason, S., Arner, S., Breivik, H., Heiskanen, T., Kalso, E., Kongsgaard, U.E., Sjogren, P., Strang, P., Bach, F.W. and Jensen, T.S. (2005) Breakthrough pain in malignant and non-malignant diseases: a review of prevalence, characteristics and mechanisms. *European Journal of Pain*, **9**(2), 195–206.

Tucker, K.L. (2004) Medico-legal case report and commentary: inadequate pain management in the context of terminal cancer. The case of Lester Tomlinson. *Pain Medicine*, **5**(2), 214–28.

Watt-Watson, J., Stevens, B., Garfinkel, P., Streiner, D. and Gallop, R. (2001) Relationship between nurses' pain knowledge and pain management outcomes for their postoperative cardiac patients. *Journal of Advanced Nursing*, **36**(4), 535–45.

Williams A.C.C. (2006) *Recommended Guidelines for Pain Management Programmes (Provisional)*. The British Pain Society. Available at <*http://www.britishpainsociety.org*>, accessed 07.07.2006.

Won, A.B., Lapane, K.L., Vallow, S., Schein, J., Morris, J.N. and Lipitz, L.A. (2004) Persistent nonmalignant pain and analgesic prescribing patterns in elderly nursing home residents. *Journal of the American Geriatric Society*, **52**(6), 867–74.

World Health Organization (1996) *Cancer Pain Relief*. WHO, Geneva.

Yong, H., Gibson, S.J., Horne, D.J. and Helme, R.D. (2001) Development of a pain attitudes questionnaire to assess Stoicism and cautiousness for possible age differences. *Journal of Gerontology*, **56B**(5), 279–84.

Web sites

Action on Pain (a UK national charity dedicated to providing support and advice for people who are affected by chronic pain): <*http://www.action-on-pain.co.uk/*>

British Pain Society (a multidisciplinary professional organization): <*http://www.britishpainsociety.org*>

International Association for the Study of Pain: <*http://www.iasp-pain.org*>

Oxford Pain Internet Site: <*http://www.jr2.ox.ac.uk/bandolier/booth/painpag/index.html*>

Pain Concern (a UK charity providing information and support for pain sufferers, those who care for them and about them): <*http://www.painconcern.org.uk*>

Pain Relief Foundation (a UK charity which funds research into the causes and treatment of human chronic pain and is concerned with education of doctors and nurses in pain management): <*http://www.painrelieffoundation.org.uk*>

Cancer pain in elderly people in palliative care settings

7

Paula Smith

Introduction

The incidence of cancer rises with age, and 64% of all diagnosed cases in the UK are in people who are over 65 years of age (Cancer Research UK, 2006). One of the most feared symptoms associated with cancer is pain, and indeed research indicates that 70–90% of people with advanced cancer experience chronic pain (Portenoy and Lesage, 2001). This is particularly likely in the terminal or end stages of the cancer journey. Pain is therefore an important symptom to consider when caring for older people with cancer. Like many industrialized countries, the United Kingdom has an ageing population (Office of National Statistics, 2006), so the likelihood is that the number of people who experience cancer in old age will increase. The purpose of this chapter is to consider the issues and management of cancer pain in an older population, and to suggest ways in which an understanding of these issues might influence nursing care.

How is cancer pain addressed in palliative care settings?

Pain in cancer is a common symptom, and pain relief was one of the central reasons behind the founding of the modern hospice movement (Clark, 2000) by Dame Cicely Saunders, and the development of the total pain concept (Clark, 1999). A core focus of the early work of the hospice movement was the relief of symptoms, and today specialist palliative care services (SPCS) have developed their ability to assess and treat the pain experienced in terminal illness, particularly in cancer care. With modern treatments and therapies cancer pain can now be controlled for most, but not all, patients (Doyle *et al.*, 2005). Despite this, a number of factors can contribute to inadequate pain control, including a lack of adequate education of physicians and other health professionals, and a generalized fear of addiction to strong opioids by both professionals and patients (WHO Expert Committee Report, 1990).

The total pain concept – the patient experience

Dame Cecily Saunders believed, based on her systematic attention to patient stories, that pain was more than just a single phenomenon (Clark, 1999). Rather, pain was experienced at a number of different levels. The **total pain concept** therefore considers the physical, social, emotional and spiritual components of the pain experience (Clark, 1999).

The total pain concept was further developed by Twycross (1997; Twycross and Wilcock, 2002) and captures a range of issues in each of the four domains related to the total pain concept:

- Within the **physical dimension** there is a need to consider the description of the pain, other concurrent symptoms caused by the illness or disease, and unwanted effects resulting from treatments. For older people this will necessarily include information about any potential other illness that might also affect the individual's perception of pain and response to it.

- In the **social dimension** there is a need to consider family roles, financial factors, friendships and isolation. Again for older people there may be particular concerns that are likely to have an effect, such as issues around caring for another person or pet.

- In the **psychological dimension** Twycross and Wilcock (2002) suggest that feelings, coping strategies and previous adjustments to loss may be important in understanding the nature of an older person's response to pain. Thus, if someone has dealt with pain in the past they may have developed adaptive coping strategies for coping with chronic pain.

- Finally, in the **spiritual dimension** a consideration of the meaning and beliefs about illness, perception of the past and future and issues around faith may have an important contribution to make to understanding and experiencing pain.

It is for these reasons that specialist palliative care approaches have developed a multiprofessional approach in order to adequately address the multidimensional nature of pain and suffering in end-of-life care.

The total pain concept highlights the personal and subjective nature of pain, which goes beyond the merely physical or biological phenomenon (Paz and Seymour, 2004). It is important therefore that during the assessment process note is taken of the experience, quality and duration of the pain in order to be able to quantify its severity and to contribute to a clinical diagnosis of its cause. Particularly in palliative care, the existential or spiritual suffering experienced may have a strong impact on the perception of pain by the patient and their family and carers.

It is therefore important that this aspect of the total pain concept is considered during the assessment of the pain experienced (Brant, 2003).

Learning point

Read around the total pain concept and identify some questions that you would ask a patient in order to address this concept in your assessment process.

Cancer pain

Cancer pain is a complex pain that requires a multidisciplinary approach (Camaioni *et al.*, 1997). It might present as either an acute or chronic pain syndrome and may or may not be associated with the tumour (Pargeon and Hailey, 1999). Recognition of the particular pain syndrome being experienced by the patient can improve the knowledge of the underlying cause, and results in more appropriate and specific therapy or interventions.

Acute pain is short in duration and resolves when the injury heals (McDonald, 1999). The physiological changes associated with this type of pain will often result in increased anxiety and agitation, which may be exacerbated in older people, particularly if they are cognitively impaired (McDonald, 1999). Within cancer acute pain flare-ups may be caused by diagnostic or therapeutic interventions, such as bone marrow biopsy, tumour embolization, intravenous or intraperitoneal infusions, or acute postradiation proctocolitis (Paz and Seymour, 2004). In addition, some people with generally well-controlled pain may experience **breakthrough pain**, which requires prompt assessment and treatment.

Chronic pain is of longer duration, typically more than six months (McDonald, 1999). Tumour-related somatic pain results from tissue or bone injury, caused for example by neoplastic invasion of bone, joint, muscle or connective tissue (Paz and Seymour, 2004). The spine is the most common site of bone metastases (Portenoy and Lesage, 2001), resulting in potentially devastating neurological damage. A patient's complaint of back pain should therefore be assessed fully, as it may indicate a potential for spinal cord compression (Portenoy and Lesage, 2001). It is essential that early diagnosis and treatment of potential problems be made in these situations.

Visceral pain occurring in organs such as kidney, stomach or liver may result in obstruction, infiltration or compression. If this happens in the nerve, plexus or dorsal roots ganglion it cause **neuropathic pain** (Paz and Seymour, 2004). Such syndromes are highly variable in patient reports and a variety of terms, such as burning or tingling, may be used to describe them (Portenoy and Lesage, 2001).

Iatrogenic pain may result from treatment such as chemotherapy or radiotherapy. Frequently patients complain of general feelings of malaise and flu-like symptoms, although some somatic pain can occur (Portenoy and Lesage, 2001). These symptoms can mimic tumour-related pain and if they are noted it is therefore important to exclude recurrence of the cancer. Most post-treatment pain is neuropathic and may be a result of nerve damage. For example, radiation-induced fibrosis can damage peripheral nerves and may sometimes cause symptoms months or years after treatment (Paz and Seymour, 2004).

Multidimensional assessment

The assessment and management of cancer pain in older adults needs to take account of the multidimensional nature of the pain experience. Simply asking an older person if they have or are experiencing pain may not be an adequate method of identifying the level and intensity of the pain experience. Krishnasamy (2001) believes that one of the nurse's greatest challenges in pain management is to consider the individual's experience of pain, and to understand the factors outside the purely physical that impinge on this. She identifies a number of questions that can be used to evaluate and assess the experience of pain from the individual's perspective. These questions focus on the patient's perspective of when they were first ill, how family and friends reacted, what makes any pain better, fears for the future, and how life plans may have been altered (Krishnasamy, 2001). This results in information about how the patient perceives the pain and the impact this is having. Such information may be particularly important in caring for older people, as they may be reluctant to share such experiences if they feel this will hold up busy health-care professionals with their 'trivial worries'. Alternatively they may believe that pain and its consequent losses are to be expected and that they should just put up with things.

A comprehensive assessment should therefore include aspects relating to the past pain history and interventions, description and location of the pain, timing of onset, intensity, any relieving or aggravating scales, and the impact the pain has on the patient's activities (McDonald, 1999). For cognitively impaired older people it may also be important to note any pain behaviours that differ from the normal behaviours of the patient, such as increased agitation, grimacing, restlessness, or protection of a painful limb (Turk and Okifuji, 2001).

While it is important to understand the person's perspective, it is also essential to measure the severity of the pain experienced objectively, in order to be able to evaluate any therapeutic interventions. Numerous tools are available to aid health professionals in this assessment. In one study the simple use of an assessment scale greatly increased the frequency of pain diagnosis in elderly nursing home residents (Kamel *et al.*, 2001). When trying to determine the intensity of the pain, visual analogue scales have been found to be useful for older people. Whichever assessment tool is chosen it is important that it is used systematically and is understandable to the patient. Furthermore, once pain has been identified it is important that its intensity and duration are re-assessed regularly, particularly if the patient has been reluctant to discuss their pain while demonstrating clear pain-related behaviours.

Learning point

Look at the discussion of pain assessment scales in Chapter 4. Which scale do you think would be most appropriate for use in your area?

The family in palliative care

The philosophy of palliative care considers the family to be integral to the care of the patient. This is significant when considering pain relief as the family are most likely to be present when the patient experiences pain, and may also play an important part in the management of this symptom. In particular, some pain behaviours may result in a secondary gain for the patient in terms of increased attention or an excuse to avoid some activities (Gloth, 2001). This needs to be restructured so that secondary gain (e.g. increased attention) is associated with pain relief rather than pain behaviours.

The extent to which family and patients agree about levels and intensity of the pain experience is variable, and family members will often overestimate the degree of pain in comparison with the patient's own reports. However, congruence between patient and family dyads about the controllability of pain was found by Riley-Doucet (2005) to have a positive influence on the family pain control outcomes. Therefore it is important that while assessing an individual patients' pain the perception of close family members are taken into account, as this may improve the efficacy of any proposed treatments.

What are the issues for older people?

A number of important issues relating to cancer pain and the older population are highlighted in the literature. These are expectations of pain in later life; co-morbidity; lack of access to SPCS; compliance with pharmacological treatments; and age-related alterations in drug disposition. These multiple barriers may result in older people being at an increased risk of experiencing uncontrolled pain (Maxwell, 2000).

Expectations of pain in later life

Older people often expect pain as part of their everyday life and experience, and often display a stoical acceptance of this. People may have developed a number of strategies for themselves that reduce or limit the pain they experience, and this is applied to the new pain experience of cancer. For example, someone who has experienced arthritic pain for a number of years is likely to have developed a number of personal coping strategies to deal with it, such as limiting painful movement, using a hot-water bottle or cold compress on affected joints, or routinely taking mild analgesics.

Co-morbidity

One of the greatest difficulties in caring for older people with cancer is the likelihood that the individual will be suffering from more than one condition at any one time. In addition to the signs and symptoms of the cancer, it is highly probable that the older person will also have experience of a chronic or long-term condition such as arthritis, diabetes, heart failure or Alzheimer's. These conditions may make it more difficult to assess the impact that the cancer or cancer treatment may have on the experience and perception of the older person's pain.

Lack of access to specialist palliative care services

There are discrepancies in the extent to which older people have access to the expert support of SPCS. Despite the increased incidence and mortality rates of older people with cancer (Cancer Research UK, 2005) they are less likely to access in-patient care than younger patients (Addington-Hall, 2004). In the Regional Study of Care for the Dying, Addington-Hall, Altmann and McCarthy (1998) found that patients under 85 years of age were almost three times more likely to have received hospice in-patient care than those over this age. This is perhaps surprising, when requirements for pain management appear to be similar to those for younger patients (Stein and Miech, 1993). Overall, however, there is little evidence in the literature about how the prevalence, perception and control of symptoms varies with age, and this is an area worthy of further investigation (Addington-Hall, 2004).

Concordance with pharmacological treatments

Many older people view pharmacological treatments as a last resort, particularly if there is an expectation that pain is a normal part of the ageing and disease process. In addition, they may be reluctant to take strong analgesia and in particular opioids because of their perceived addictive nature, or a perception that they will result in a lack of awareness of what is going on, or an early death.

Age-related alterations in drug disposition

The World Health Organization has developed a staged approach to pain relief (WHO 1990). This commences with the introduction of mild analgesia and progresses towards strong opioids. The difficulty when treating older people is that their metabolism may affect the dosage and reactions to some drugs that are routinely prescribed for cancer pain. Furthermore, the side effects of some of these drugs may be experienced more severely by older people and this may contribute to their reluctance to take such medication. In elderly patients careful, tailored management of pharmacological therapy is required (Camaioni et al, 1997).

Learning point

Consider a patient in your area with cancer. Which if any of the above issues are relevant to their experience of cancer pain and pain relief?

Management of cancer pain in elderly people in palliative care

The management of cancer pain in older people can be pharmacological, non-pharmacological or a combination of the two.

Pharmalogical approach

WHO (1990) has created an easy-to-use three-step analgesic ladder for use in the management of pain. The method is used extensively in palliative care and comprises a stepwise approach to ensuring adequate pain relief. It recommends that analgesia should be given by the mouth, by the clock, by the ladder, and then reviewed (Paz and Seymour, 2004). This approach ensures that adequate pain relief is delivered regularly and in increasing strength: from non-opioid analgesia, to weak opioid analgesia, to strong opioid analgesia. Most importantly, this is a framework of conceptual principles which is practical to implement. Pain treatment can be commenced at the first, second or third step according to the pain intensity. Morphine is the opioid of first choice in cancer pain relief (Hanks *et al.*, 2001).

Although the WHO approach has been extremely successful in controlling pain in many patients with cancer, there are some considerations that are important when working with older people. Some older people receive inadequate pain relief, as practitioners are reluctant to prescribe opioid drugs because of their different absorption rates and problems with toxicity. In a study by Bernabei *et al.* (1998) of older cancer patients in daily pain 16% were prescribed drugs at WHO level 1 and 32% at WHO level 2, but only 26% received morphine (a level 3 drug). In addition, patients over the age of 85 years were less likely to receive strong opiates than those aged 65–74 years. In general the rule for pharmacological dosing is to 'begin low and go slowly' (Gloth, 2001, p. 197).

Non-pharmacological approach

Given the concerns about side effects and increased toxicity in older people, the use of non-pharmacological approaches to treatment may be particularly appropriate. This may include the application of heat (stimulating the production of endogenous opioids) or cold (suppressing the release of products of tissue damage) to the pain area (Gloth, 2001). In a similar way, transcutaneous electrical nerve stimulation (TENS) and acupuncture have proved to be effective in reducing the conscious experience of pain (Carroll and Bowsher, 1993). Physical therapy, maintaining mobility and positioning the patient appropriately have all been used effectively in moderate pain (McDonald, 1999). When pain is severe these approaches may be used as an adjunct to analgesic therapy.

In some cases it is not possible to reduce the pain and therefore enhancing a person's coping skills or helping them to evaluate their pain in a more positive way is important. Cognitive behavioural therapy (CBT) has been found to improve quality of life and mood in cancer patients and this is considered a successful outcome (Carroll and Bowsher, 1993). Similarly, relaxation techniques may help to reduce muscular tension and stress and anxiety (Horn and Mufano, 1997), and act as a distractor to the pain. More work is needed in this area to find the efficacy of these approaches with an older population; however, given the reluctance of some people and health professionals to use pharmacological approaches it may prove a beneficial avenue to consider.

Concordance with pharmacological therapy

Although many of the drugs recommended by the WHO analgesic ladder may be appropriately given to older people, it is recognized that some may have differing effects and resultant toxicity for this group of patients. In addition, the use of strong opioid drugs can result in common side effects (e.g. constipation) that can be more distressing to an older person than the original pain experienced.

For this reason compliance and concordance with recommended pharmacological treatments may be difficult to achieve, without a detailed assessment of the presenting pain and an adequate discussion about the recommended management. This will necessarily need to include information about potential side effects (constipation) and ways to reduce this side effect (regular prescription of laxative).

Other treatments

Alternative treatments and therapies may be more acceptable to older people than traditional pharmacological approaches, particularly for mild or moderate pain control. Such treatments may include simply changing the patient's position if they have been resting in one place for a long period of time, or the use of external sources of relief such as hot or cold compresses, or electrical stimulation of the nerves.

Recommendations for practice

It is clear that a number of recommendations for practice emerge from an understanding of the issues surrounding the assessment, treatment and evaluation of cancer pain in older people within palliative care settings. Guidelines for good practice will assist in this process and should be referred to when considering the management of pain.

Assessment and management

The total pain concept alerts us to the multidimensional nature of the pain experience. Particularly in cancer and palliative care, the spiritual and existential dimension of suffering may influence the perception of the pain experience and the degree to which an older person feels able to control this. Previous experience of seeing others in pain with cancer may also influence their expectations, and it is important that these factors are considered and discussed if they are not to have undue influence on current treatment and help-seeking by the patient and their family. Health-care professionals therefore need to use the tools and treatment recommendations in their own clinical decisions about the best treatment and efficacy for each individual case.

Roles of the multidisciplinary team

The multidisciplinary nature of palliative care provision characterizes adequate pain control. Combined pharmacological and non-pharmacological approaches can be used successfully to enhance the pain management of older people within palliative care. For example, the physiotherapist may be able to advise on appropriate exercise and movement, which will complement the pharmacological approaches being used. The introduction of alternative therapies such as aromatherapy and relaxation may also be important in helping individuals to reassess or be distracted from their pain experience, and thus improve their overall quality of life.

SPCS intervention

Despite the number of older people who experience cancer, their ability to access SPCS intervention is limited. It is therefore important that general health-care professionals are aware of the special factors that need to be considered when assessing and managing an older person with cancer pain, and the time points when it may be appropriate to seek more specialist help.

One particularly important factor is the development of a good working relationship with the patient and their family or carers. When there is open and honest communication about any potential pain that may be experienced, it is possible for a detailed assessment and treatment plan to be developed. This will have the advantage of ensuring that the patient's perspective is fully considered, including the social, spiritual and physical dimensions of the pain and suffering that may be experienced.

Full use of the WHO three-step ladder for pain control, including opioids, should be considered, bearing in mind the particular difficulties that older people may experience. With careful introduction, explanations and information it is possible for older people's cancer pain to be successfully managed, even if a number of additional diseases are present.

Conclusion

The incidence of cancer increases in older age. Pain is a common feature of cancer and therefore the number of older people who are and will be experiencing cancer pain is set to rise over time. Despite this, older people are less likely to be able to access SPCS. This may influence the management of their pain experience and it is therefore important that general health-care professionals are aware of the need to assess the total pain experience sensitively and accurately, in order to manage the older person's pain appropriately.

The concept of the total pain experience is important within palliative care, as this takes into account the physical, spiritual, social and psychological aspects of an individual's pain. There are a number of factors that might make older people reluctant to share their pain and therefore it is important that health-care professionals are able to assess both the intensity of pain and wider factors that might influence the experience.

Management of the total pain experience may involve the use of both pharmacological and non-pharmacological approaches. It is important that pharmacological approaches are appropriate for the pain intensity experienced, but are titrated carefully to reduce the consequence of side effects and toxicity. Non-pharmacological approaches may be more acceptable to older people for mild to moderate pain, and may be used effectively as an adjunct to stronger analgesia and opioids in severe pain.

Learning point

Assessment of pain needs to be done sensitively.

Summary

- Elderly people with cancer experience unrecognized and unacknowledged pain.
- Multiple pathologies make recognition of pain difficult in palliative care settings.
- Older people are less likely to have access to specialist palliative care services therefore it is important for general health care providers to be aware of the special needs of older people.
- Non-pharmacological treatments for mild to moderate pain may be preferred by older people.

References

Addington-Hall, J. (2004) Referral patterns and access to care, in *Palliative Care Nursing: Principles and Evidence For Practice* (eds S. Payne, J. Seymour and C. Ingleton), Open University Press, Buckingham.

Addington-Hall, J., Altmann, D. and McCarthy, M. (1998) Who gets hospice in-patient care?. *Social Science and Medicine*, **46**(8), 1011–16.

Bernabei, R., Gambassi, G., Lapane, K., Landi, F., Gatsonis, C., Dunlop, R., Lipsitz, L., Steel, K. and Mor, V. (1998) Management of pain in elderly patients with cancer. SAGE study group. Systematic assessment of geriatric drug use via epidemiology. *Journal of the American Medical Association*, **279**(23), 1877–82.

Brant, J. (2003) Pain management, in *Palliative Care Nursing: A Guide to Practice*, 2nd edn (eds M. O'Connor and S. Aranda), Ausumed Publications, Melbourne, VIC.

Camaioni, D., Evangelista, M., Mascaro, A., Bosco, M., Stancanelli, V., Montagna, A. and Annetta, M.G. (1997) Pain therapy in elderly cancer patients. *Rays*, **22**(1), 47–52.

Cancer Research UK (2005) *CancerStats Mortality – UK*. Available at: <*http://info.cancerresearchuk.org/cancerstats/mortality/?a=5441*>

Cancer Research UK (2006) *CancerStats Incidence – UK*. Available at: <*http://info.cancerresearchuk.org/cancerstats/incidence/?a=5441*>, accessed September 2006.

Carroll, D. and Bowsher, D. (1993) *Pain Management and Nursing Care*. Butterworth-Heinemann, Oxford.

Clark, D. (1999) 'Total pain', disciplinary power and the body in the work of Cicely Saunders 1958–67. *Social Science and Medicine*, **49**(6), 727–36.

Clark, D. (2000) *Cicely Saunders, Founder of the Hospice Movement: Selected Letters 1959–1999*. Oxford University Press, Oxford.

Doyle, D., Hanks, G., Cherny, N. and Claman, K. (2005) *Oxford Textbook of Palliative Medicine*, 3rd edn. Oxford University Press, Oxford.

Gloth, F.M. (2001) Pain management in older adults: prevention and treatment. *J ournal of the American Geriatrics Society*, **49**, 188–99.

Hanks, G.W., Conno, F. and Cherny, N. *et al.* (2001) Expert working group of the research network of the European Association for Palliative Care – morphine and alternative opioids in cancer pain: the EAPC recommendations. *British Journal of Cancer*, **84**(5), 587–93.

Horn, S. and Mufano, M. (1997) *Pain: Theory, Research and Intervention*. Open University Press, Buckingham.

Kamel, H.K., Phlavan, M., Maledgoudarzi, B., Gogel, P. and Morley, J.E. (2001) Utilizing pain assessment scales increases the frequency of diagnosing pain among elderly nursing home residents. *Journal of Pain and Symptom Management*, **21**(6), 450–5.

Krishnasamy, M. (2001) Pain, in *Cancer Nursing Care in Context* (eds J. Corner and C. Bailey), Blackwell Science, Oxford.

McDonald, M. (1999) Assessment and management of cancer pain in the cognitively impaired elderly. *Geriatric Nursing,* **20**(5), 249–54.

Maxwell, T. (2000) Cancer pain management in the elderly. *Geriatric Nursing,* **21**(3), 158–63.

Office of National Statistics (2006) *Population Ageing.* Available at: <*http://www. statistics.gov.uk/cci/nugget.asp?id=4949*>, accessed September 2006.

Pargeon, K.L. and Hailey, B.J. (1999) Barriers to effective cancer pain management: a review of the literature. *Journal of Pain and Symptom Management,* **18**(5), 358–68.

Paz, S. and Seymour, J. (2004) Pain: theories, evaluation and management, in *Palliative Care Nursing: Principles and Evidence for Practice* (eds S. Payne, J. Seymour and C. Ingleton), Open University Press, Buckingham.

Portenoy, R.K. and Lesage, P. (2001) Management of cancer pain. The pain series. *The Lancet,* **353**(9165), 1695–700.

Riley-Doucet, C. (2005) beliefs about the controllability of pain: congruence between older adults with cancer and their family caregivers. *Journal of Family Nursing,* **11**(3), 225–41.

Stein, W.M. and Miech, R.P. (1993) Cancer pain in the elderly hospice patients. *Journal of Pain and Symptom Management,* **8**(7), 474–82.

Turk, D.C. and Okifuji, A. (2001) Assessment of patients' reporting of pain: an integrated perspective. The pain series. *The Lancet,* **353**(9166), 1784–8.

Twycross, R. (1997) *Oral Morphine in Advanced Cancer,* 3rd edn. Beaconsfield Publishers, Beaconsfield.

Twycross, R., and Wilcock, A. (2002) *Symptom Management in Advanced Cancer,* 3rd edn. Radcliffe Medical Press, Oxford.

World Health Organization (1990) *Cancer Pain Relief and Palliative Care.* Technical Report Series 804. WHO, Geneva.

Care homes and other settings

8

Pat Schofield

Introduction

Adults are living longer and are surviving episodes of acute illness as a result of health-care advancements. As a result, health-care professionals will encounter older adults in every clinical setting. The issue to be considered is whether or not these adults need to be treated any differently, or do we simply adapt our usual pain management strategies to meet their needs? The aim of this chapter is to discuss the range of settings in which older people may be cared for, and to identify and explore the issues around pain management for this group. Some clinical examples of experiences will be presented and a case will be made for multidisciplinary/multimodal management.

Pain is the most common symptom of disease and the most common complaint reported to doctors. However, chronic pain can present a perplexing problem for doctors, which has resulted in the widespread acceptance of the need for specialized chronic pain clinics in developed countries (Ferrell, 1991). Although the consequences of chronic pain are well documented, issues relating to chronic pain in the older population are less so. For example, Melding (1991) found that of the 4000 papers published annually related to pain, less than 1% focused on pain in the older population; and a review of 8 geriatric textbooks showed that they contained only 18 out of 5000 pages on pain. The specific problems of pain management in older people have only begun to be addressed systematically over the last decade. Within the United Kingdom, the recent National Service Frameworks for older people (Department of Health, 2001) have highlighted the need to address chronic pain in the older age groups. A presentation at the International Association for the Study of Pain conference (Gibson, 2002) suggested that it is time for clinicians to 'grasp the nettle' and provide services tailored to meet the needs of older people as the numbers in pain are increasing and will represent two thirds of the pain population worldwide by 2020. It is estimated that 25–50% of community-dwelling adults are suffering from pain that reaches a significantly high level at last some of the time (American Geriatric Society, 1998). One of the most common pain syndromes in this group is musculoskeletal pain (Kahana *et al.*, 1997), although other researchers highlight common sites including low back pain (Andersson *et al.*, 1993) or joint pain (Mobiliy *etal.*, 1994). A study by Elliott, Smith and Penny (1999) highlighted that the incidence of chronic pain in the community significantly increased in the over-65 age group in their random sample of 5036 patients in the Grampian region of Scotland.

In addition, it has been suggested that 45–80% of the care-home population are experiencing pain (Fox, Raina and Jadad, 1999). The most common sources of pain within this group are found to be low back pain, arthritis and previous fractures (Ferrell, Ferrell and Osterwell, 1990). Furthermore, Senstaken and King (1993) highlighted that 40–50% of care-home residents were taking analgesic drugs but that older age appears to be a risk factor for inadequate pain management (Cleeland *et al.*, 1994). This evidence suggests that a more creative pain management protocol is needed for this group, focusing more on multidimensional management.

In terms of rehabilitation, several pain-producing conditions have been highlighted. For example, post-stroke pain is considered to be one of the most unrecognized sequelae of stroke (Benrud-Larson and Wegener, 2000). **Central post-stroke pain** (CRPS), which is constant and severe, develops in approximately 8% of patients in the year following their stroke (Anderson *et al.*, 1995). Musculoskeletal pain following stroke occurs in 33–40% of patients (Anderson *et al.*, 1995) and most patients with hemiparesis develop shoulder pain in the affected limb. Another very significant pain problem seen in older adults in rehabilitation areas is **phantom limb pain** (PLP) after an amputation. Pain occurs in the residual limb in approximately 50% of patients (Hill, 1999) and PLP can occur in 50–80% of amputees (Davis, 1993).

Postoperative care of older adults presents many challenges to health-care professionals. Problems highlighted are related to communication (Bergh *et al.*, 2005), fears of prescribing and using strong opioids (Ferrell, 1996) and a number of other barriers that have been highlighted within the literature (McCaffery and Pasero, 1995). Such barriers relate to beliefs held by older people themselves, their relatives and caregivers and include fears of bothering caregivers, a belief that older people get used to pain and fears around addiction. Opiophobia has been highlighted in the literature as a major barrier to prescribing and taking opioids (Morgan, 1985).

Learning point

In the area where you work, what are the views of staff regarding older adults in your care?

Problems with chronic pain in older people

In November 1990, a care-home owner in the USA was found negligent in failing to give adequate pain management to a resident with prostate cancer (Shapiro, 1994). The lawsuit focused on the responsibility of health-care providers to provide adequate pain medication and concluded that this failure had caused the resident undue physical pain, suffering and mental anguish. Such events have highlighted the need to focus attention on the effective management of pain in the care-home population, which according to the epidemiological evidence mentioned earlier is often inadequate.

Physiological changes?

Although there is an increasing literature on the management of pain in older people, there are still a number of concerns. For example, it has been suggested that age-related changes may result in complex alterations in the processing of pain through the nervous system (Melzack and Wall, 1990; Melding, 1991). Examples of this are often seen when patients are admitted with silent myocardial infarctions (Bayer, Bresloff and Curley, 1986) and abdominal catastrophes (Bender, 1989). However, despite the relevance of these studies, which have been questioned in practice (Agency for Healthcare Policy and Research, 1992), there is still a widespread belief that ageing decreases pain perception. An alternative point of view is that older people get used to pain (Harkins, Price and Braith, 1989).

Getting used to pain?

It has been suggested that 80% of people over the age of 65 suffer from at least one chronic illness (Harkins, Price and Braith, 1989; Kane, Ouslander and Abrass, 1989) and many of these illnesses are associated with pain. For example, according to Valkenburg (1988) 30% of men and 53% of women over the age of 55 experience peripheral joint pains. Blomqvist (2003), in her study of pain in a group of 150 older people, found a range of potentially painful conditions including falls, leg ulcers, degenerative joints and cancer; many of these conditions were well known and visible, yet the management of pain in this group was poor. Yates and Fentiman (1995) also found that care-home residents themselves accepted that they had to put up with the pain and did not expect it to be managed. Blomqvist (2003) found that residents were reluctant even to report pain, as they perceived staff to be uninterested and unwilling to provide any pain relief. Clearly, the literature appears to suggest that both staff and residents perceive pain to be a natural part of ageing and that pain management is not seen as a priority.

Assessment

There have been major developments in the field of pain assessment, in particular the introduction of the McGill Pain Questionnaire as a multidimensional pain tool (Herr and Mobily, 1991). Many reasons have been given for why pain assessment in older people is poor (Closs *et al.*, 2004). For example, it has been suggested that some older people accept that they have to live with pain: they have limited belief that the pain can be eliminated, or they may fear medications and their subsequent side effects (American Geriatric Society, 2002). Where assessment scales have been used, some success has been reported with the visual analogue scale, the verbal descriptors scale and the faces scale (Horgas, 2003). However, as suggested by Closs *et al.* (2004) in their study examining the use of pain assessment scales, some residents may be prevented from using these scales because of hearing or visual difficulties. Furthermore, attempting to apply pain scales for residents with cognitive impairments can also be challenging for staff. However, there have been some major breakthroughs recently, with a behavioural pain scale being introduced in Australia (Abbey *et al.*, 2004) and the DOLOPLUS scale (Chapiro, 2001) in France. These scales have been specifically designed to measure pain in older people who are unable to communicate their pain, and the authors report on research that successfully utilizes these scales in practice (see Chapter 4).

Management

When an older adult complains of mild to moderate pain, many health-care providers are content to do nothing (Roberto and Gold, 2001). The alternative appears to be a pharmacological approach. However, a high incidence of sensitivity to medications is reported. For example, non-steroidal anti-inflammatory drugs (NSAIDs) cause a high incidence of gastrointestinal bleeding and the use of opioid analgesics is also controversial (Popp and Portenoy, 1996). Lovheim *et al.* (2006) found that 56.7% of their sample of care-home residents were in pain (3724) and only 27.9% of the residents were receiving analgesia. Yet 72.7% of staff thought that the residents were being treated for their pain, demonstrating a serious lack of awareness amongst care-home staff of the types and nature of pharmacological pain interventions.

A recent systematic review of published articles (Fox, Raina and Jadad, 1999) looking at pain in the older population found that of 91 potential papers studied only 3 evaluated the effectiveness of interventions for the treatment of pain in this group. One study investigated relaxation (Moye and Hanlon, 1996), one investigated humorous films (Adams and McGuire, 1986) and the third investigated exercise (Miller and LeLieuvre, 1982). Fox, Raina and Jadad (1999) considered that further research was needed, focusing on investigation of both pharmacological and non-pharmacological strategies.

A more recent review by Roberto and Gold (2001) covered 3745 articles and noted that there was a dearth of literature relating to issues and concerns of older people with chronic pain, and therefore recommended that future studies should focus on preferred strategies of older people. This is supported by the recommendations of Ferrell and Ferrell (1996) who suggest that strategies for the management of pain in older adults should encompass non-pharmacological approaches that enhance quality of life and reduce the potential for unpleasant side effects, while also exploring the use of the three-step analgesic ladder (World Health Organization, 1990) as a pharmacological guideline for this group (see Chapter 7).

Education

Lack of education of health-care staff is often cited as a major causal factor in poor pain management (Cowan et al., 2003). Many authors have suggested that doctors and nurses lack the education necessary to make an informed choice regarding the most appropriate pain management strategies (Cowan et al., 2003). Some recommendations for improvements have been made (Cowan et al., 2003) and in recent years some of these recommendations have been taken on board and the development of pain services has addressed many of the education needs, along with Pain Society guidance on minimal educational requirements. Training programmes such as the English National Board N53 or masters programmes have been introduced. (Although the ENB no longer exists, the pain course has been incorporated into diploma or degree programmes.) But recent work suggests that care-home staff are still not adequately educated about the principles of pain management (Allcock, McGarry and Elkan, 2002). Whether this is because the homes are in the independent sector and so staff do not have access to programmes within acute NHS trusts, or whether they do not have the resources to release staff, is unclear. Alternatively, it could be that most care-home staff are not registered nurses and there are few educational programmes of specifically designed for them. If this is the case, there is a desperate need to provide such programmes tailored to the needs of health-care workers who have front-line access to older people and could potentially offer a range of pain management strategies. However, the Department of Health has funded palliative care education for community nurses and in some areas this has been offered to care-home staff.

Assets

Yonan and Wegener (2003) suggest that although there are barriers to the management of pain in older adults, this population also has many assets that help them to cope with pain. For example, Bengston *et al.* (1985) showed that self-esteem increases with age, which helps older people to retain their sense of self-worth in the face of many losses. Furthermore, Erikson *et al.* (1986) suggest that older adults have achieved a sense of meaning in their lives, which helps them to cope with stressful life events. Research by Baltes (1991) highlighted that older adults can compensate for age-related losses by modifying their goals and aspirations to fit current life circumstances. Thus, older adults appear to have coping strategies for dealing with pain that are similar to those employed by their younger counterparts and equally effective (Keefe and Williams, 1990).

Although the results of research into pain tolerance in this group are still inconclusive, some suggest that older adults have a greater tolerance for pain than their younger counterparts (Galgliese *et al.*, 1999) and therefore have a higher pain threshold. Researchers also speculate that older adults expect pain as part of getting older (Cook and Thomas, 1994; Riley *et al.*, 2000). This is also consistent with the finding that older adults report diminished emotional responses to pain, such as depression, anxiety and fear, and exhibit less pain behaviour than their younger counterparts (Riley *et al.*, 2000). All of these can be useful considerations when dealing with older adults and helping them to develop coping strategies.

Ongoing research

There is a lot of recent research into issues surrounding pain in the care-home population. For example, Closs *et al.* (2004) investigated the use of pain assessment tools for cognitively impaired adults and Allcock *et al.* (2002) investigated the attitudes of staff towards residents in pain. A number of studies have focused on the assessment of pain, with a particular emphasis on patients with cognitive impairment (Simons and Malabar, 1995) or Alzheimer's disease (Hurley *et al.*, 1992). The author has recently completed a study investigating residents' own perspectives of their pain and their preferred pain management strategies in a small study in one district. This had led to the development of a distance learning package for care-home staff to improve their knowledge of pain, pain assessment and management.

Comments made by residents when asked to discuss their pain

Reluctance to report pain, acceptance and low expectations

Mrs Jones (82 years) mentioned that she had a 'problem' with her neck but that it did not cause her any pain. When asked if she had arthritis she then commented that she did have arthritis in her knees, hips and joints, which were very painful, but said, 'I don't like to complain, the staff are very busy'.

Mr Smith (77 years) attends the pain clinic. When asked to talk about his pain he said:

> I have been in pain in my spine, over 20 years now . . . They give me injections every six months, but they don't help, not even for a couple of days. I don't tell the staff, as they would send me back in hospital, I am not going back in there, so I don't let them know.

Mrs Green (80 years) stated that although it hurts, 'It's not enough to grumble about, I don't like to complain'. She described her arthritis pain as not being 'real pain   like childbirth – more like a toothache, you can live with it, this is what happens when you get to my age'.

Many of the residents commented that the pain woke them at night, but they did not want to disturb the night staff. Comments included:

> I do not like to complain to the night staff they are very, busy, so I just lay there and hope that I can get back to sleep – I don't sleep much anyway. (Mrs Jones)
> I don't sleep very well at night, every time I move it wakes me up. (Mrs Smith)

Other comments included:

> It's not unbearable, it just reminds me it's there, but there's nothing anyone can do so I don't grumble. (Mrs Brown, 68 years)
> There's nothing anyone can do to help. (Mrs Green)

I really need a new set of legs and they can't do that for me, so I just get on with it. (Mrs Davis, 66 years)

What can you do, I just have to make the most of what I have, at least I can still get around. (Mr Stone, 78 years)

There's no point telling the staff, they try to help, but there's nothing they can do. (Mr Smith)

They're so busy, they haven't got time to mess around with me, there are others much worse off. (Mrs Jones)

I've had this pain for so long now, there's nothing anyone can do, I just ignore it. (Mr Stone)

Fear of chemical/pharmacological interventions

Many of the residents, particularly in the older age group (>75 years), commented that they were fearful of using chemical or pharmacological interventions and would rather manage without. When asked about taking tablets for pain, they often commented that they did not really help with the pain and they did not want anything stronger. One resident stated:

I'm living on drugs er tablets. Well, I don't know if they work, they seem to, I don't want anything stronger. (Miss Staple, 77 years)

I don't like the way they make me feel – dizzy, sleepy, all I do is sleep. (Mrs Smith)

I'm not a young man and would expect to be in pain at this age, so taking tablets is not the answer. You can live with pain, but not the way the drugs make you feel. (Mr Hand, 88 years)

Mr Good (91 years) commented that he did not like taking the drugs as they made him constipated. When asked what he did about the pain he said, 'laughing helps'. Another resident, Mrs Brown, said 'I don't take anything, unless I'm absolutely forced to. It's not good for you, to take drugs'.

Many residents appeared to take tablets only when absolutely necessary, certainly not regularly, even though they were in pain from arthritis. One resident commented that he had been prescribed ibuprofen in hospital 'so I must have arthritis, then' – as if no one had explained this too him, or he had perhaps been told and forgotten. Another resident commented that he had found the ibruprofen helped but the doctor had stopped it for some reason.

Some residents stated that they took co-codamol whenever the staff brought it to them, but they never thought to ask, they assumed the staff knew when to give it.

A further comment made was that they have 'strong willpower', as if this is to be perceived as being good. Other opinions included:

> It's no use taking drugs, they just make you feel worse, and that's all they can offer (Mr Grey, 81 years)
>
> I don't think it does you any good, taking all those tablets, they must upset you in other ways, better just to get on with the pain. (Mr Saheed, 77 years)
>
> I've never taken drugs in my life and I don't intend to start now' (Mrs Ming, 92 years)
>
> I'm taking so many tablets, I don't know what they're all for, I'm sure half of them aren't doing anything for me. (Mr Crow, 82 years)
>
> I'm sure that's why I can't keep awake all day, it's all those tablets, I'm not taking any more. (Mr Arthur, 88 years)
>
> What's the point, they don't work anyway. (Miss Sands, 74 years)

Age-related perceptions of pain

It was interesting to note that the older people appeared to be more willing to suffer with their pain and reluctant to take any analgesics. In fact they were very reluctant even to report their pain. In contrast, the residents who were more vocal about their pain were in the over-75 age group and they were willing to take some analgesics. For example, comments like the following were all made by residents in the 'older' age group:

> I'm not taking anything else, I'm already taking loads of tablets.' (Mr Smith)
>
> They don't do you any good, all those chemicals. (Mrs Ming)
>
> I'd sooner not take tablets, they make me feel worse, I like to listen to my music. (Mrs Evie)
>
> What's the point, they don't work anyway. (Mr Good)

In contrast, comments made by the younger age group (under 75) included:

> I take plenty of tablets, a few more won't make much difference. (Miss May, 68 years)
>
> I used to buy things from the chemist when I was at home, but they don't like you to do that in here, so you have to ask for them. That annoys me, why should I ask for them, I know what my pain is like, not them. (Mr Pickard, 65 years)

Lack of awareness of potential strategies for dealing with pain

Although residents appeared eager to be involved in their own pain management, they did not have any awareness of potential non-pharmacological strategies that could be available to them.

Comments included that they found a 'hot bath or shower' useful, or 'rubbing the affected area' But when asked about using heat pads or massage, they were not aware of these options. Music, distraction and television were also things that the residents stated that they found helped. None of the residents was aware of acupuncture, but one or two had occasionally used a TENS machine.

In summary, the following have emerged as key issues from conversations with to older residents about their pain:

- Lack of awareness of potential strategies for dealing with pain.
- Age-related perceptions of pain.
- Fear of chemical/pharmacological interventions.
- Reluctance to report pain.
- An acceptance that being in pain is normal.
- Low expectations for help with medical interventions.

So it is important when working in any setting that cares for older adults to take into account some of the attitudes that the older people may have about pain which, coupled with the attitudes and beliefs of health-care staff, can lead to poor pain management.

Multidisciplinary management

Learning point

Consider the members of the multidisciplinary team – who is involved in pain management within your area?

It has long been accepted that multidisciplinary pain management is the key to success, particularly in the management of chronic pain. Dealing with older adults should be no exception. As discussed in previous chapters, the impact of pain on older adults can be catastrophic in that decreased mobility, impaired ability to perform self-care, social isolation and depressed mood can result in institutionalization. The contribution of members of the multidisciplinary team in improving function, self-care and mood along with counselling and support for the taking of medication is well documented in the literature (Stuck *et al.*, 1993) and should be part of accepted care for older adults, particularly in the community.

Care at home relies principally on low-tech strategies, but the use of non-pharmacological approaches cannot be underestimated. Fears about the use of drugs, risk of side effects and potential addiction can result in non-concordance among older adults. Non-pharmacological approaches can provide more effective pain relief with less reliance on medication, fewer side effects and less clinical impairment (Mobiliy *et al.*, 1994). Unfortunately, many health-care providers perceive that older adults are reluctant to use these approaches, although this is in fact not the case. Many coping strategies such as prayer, crying and distraction have been reported to be effective in this age group (Ferrell *et al.*, 1993). This was also demonstrated earlier in some of the comments made by residents.

Social support is also important for older adults, particularly in the home. Walker *et al.* (1990) found that older adults were reassured by having someone there to 'listen' and provide encouragement and support, as opposed to providing pain management. It seems that 'caring' is once again undervalued by nurses.

The burdens borne by family members are well documented (Ferrell, 1993; Ferrell and Ferrell, 1996). Lack of sleep, distressing symptoms and work adjustment are commonly reported problems (Ferrell, 1993). The educational support of family members is essential to enable them to cope with the demands placed upon them. Ferrell (1993) demonstrated that education of family members and patients can improve pain relief. So what can the multidisciplinary team contribute to the care of older adults in the community (Table 8.1)?

There are very few multidisciplinary pain clinics specifically designed to deal with the problems of older adults. However, some authors have noted that standard pain clinics can deal with older people effectively, with some slight modification of standards. Generic treatment goals such as optimization of medication use, targets for physical activity and decreased pain are likely to be similar across the age spectrum. However, there are some age-related variations such as occupational rehabilitation and restoration of physical function that may be more relevant for the younger adults. The focus for older adults will probably encompass resuming recreational, spiritual and social interaction along with maintenance of functional independence within a community setting. Targets for reducing medication or improving physical activity may appear simple for health-care professionals, but the older adults themselves will need to be part of the planning process. It is also important to remember that older adults may be experiencing a number of co-morbidities, some of which can result in frailty that can influence

Table 8.1 The roles of the multidisciplinary team

Physician	Prescribing
	Diagnosing
	Invasive treatment options
Nurse	Caring
	Reassurance
	Education/information
	Counselling
	Support
Psychologist	Sleep management
	Stress management
	Coping strategies
Physiotherapist	Movement
	Activity
	Exercise
	Massage
	TENS
	Acupuncture
Occupational therapist	Activities of living
	Movement

participation in pain management (Corran, Helme and Gibson, 2001). It is evident, therefore, that no one specialist has all of the necessary skills to provide the support needed by older adults and their families at home.

Cognitive behavioural therapy

Cognitive behavioural therapy (CBT) is a structured psychotherapeutic approach to help individuals to develop beliefs, attitudes, thoughts and skills that enable them to modify the pain experience and thus cope more effectively. This approach has been widely accepted in the field of pain management since its introduction by Turk, Meichenbaum and Genest (1983). Such programmes offer either operant conditioning (Fordyce, 1976) or CBT interventions (Flor, Fydric and Turk, 1992). The former approach offers modification of observable behaviours and the latter modifies individuals' thoughts, feelings and behaviours. Both approaches are well documented in the literature as being successful in dealing with chronic pain in younger adults. But there has been a reluctance to use these programmes with older adults, as there may be a perception that older adults do not have the ability to be introspective or may be hampered by the presence of cognitive impairment (Yonan and Wegener, 2003). Nevertheless researchers have demonstrated that older adults are less likely to drop out of programmes (Sorkin et al., 1990) and are more likely to be able to learn self-regulation techniques such as relaxation Middaugh et al. (1991). Recent studies using CBT have demonstrated real improvements with the approach both in the reduction of anxiety (Barrowclough et al., 2001) and in the treatment of low back pain (Reid et al., 2003) as long as the older adults are cognitively intact.

It is evident that CBT is appropriate for older adults as long as some considerations are taken on board (Secker, Kazantzis and Pachana, 2004):

- Older adults can be more complicated than their younger counterparts in terms of co-morbidities, financial, interpersonal and family stressors.
- Mild cognitive impairment can be undetected and prevent the patient focusing upon the session.
- Trust and rapport can be more difficult to achieve because of the age difference.
- Memory decline can influence the ability to practise.
- Mental fatigue can occur if too much material is presented.
- Cohort-specific attitudes and stressors can influence treatment goals.
- Homework improves progress but needs to be carefully presented and not too complex.
- Frequency of attendance is influenced by transport issues.
- The teacher/student structure can seem patronizing to older adults.

Care-home settings

The final section of this chapter considers issues specifically related to the care-home setting. Within this environment live the oldest and frailest members of the population. It has been suggested that pain is more likely to be prevalent in the older population (Hicks, 2000). This may be due to the high incidence of musculoskeletal disorders, phantom limb pain, pressure ulcers, cancer and other medical conditions that can be present in this group (Ferrell, 1991). A health survey commissioned by the Department of Health (2001) did not assess for the incidence of pain, but it did demonstrate that 30% of residents in care homes were experiencing arthritis, rheumatism or problems with bones, muscles and joints, thus confirming the work of Ferrell (1991) and confirming the fact that there must be a high incidence of pain in this group.

A recent study by Won *et al.* (2004) investigated 21 380 care-home residents in the USA and demonstrated that 25% of their sample were not taking any analgesia and the most common analgesic drug in use was paracetamol. The investigators were able to conclude from this study that prescribing in the USA was suboptimal and could only be improved by education of staff.

Closs (1996) found that nurses tended to be over-cautious in the use of opioids because an exaggerated fear of side effects, particularly respiratory depression. Physicians have also been shown to have a similar fear, which has been termed **opiophobia** (Morgan, 1985). However, although older people can be more sensitive to drugs (Herr, 2002) this should not preclude them from taking opioids. Opiophobia is not restricted to staff; Brockopp *et al.* (1996) demonstrated that older people themselves were fearful of taking opioids. Similar findings have been demonstrated in our current study, with the residents commenting that they did not want to take anything stronger, or that they did not like the way the drugs made them feel. Schumacher *et al.* (2002) reported similar findings in their study which evaluated the implementation of a self-help programme in the community. Their study highlighted the strongly held conviction that medications are 'toxins' and should be avoided at all costs. This is in contrast to the study of Lumme-Sandt, Hervonen and Jylla (2000), who found with their interpretive repertoires that the older people tended to consider the use of drugs as part of everyday living: for example, getting up, having breakfast and taking their medication.

Another relevant consideration is that most of the care given to this group is delivered by unregistered practitioners, often without any training. Usually there is a limited number of registered nurses on duty, and medical support is provided by a local general practitioner. How then can effective pain control be achieved in this group? There are several issues which need to be considered.

Assessment

Issues around pain assessment have been discussed earlier in the book (Chapter 4). When dealing with any individual in pain it is important that an appropriate assessment be performed. As discussed previously, this can be hampered by increasing levels of cognitive impairment which are more likely to be present in the care-home setting. Flexibility and innovation are the key issues in enabling assessment to take place; the process requires an awareness of the available pain assessment tools for adults and adults with cognitive impairment. Furthermore, skilled and experienced health-care professionals can carry out an intuitive pain assessment based on their knowledge of the individual concerned and recognition of behavioural changes.

Attitudes and misconceptions

Much requires to be done in this area to eliminate stereotypical attitudes and beliefs related to older adults 'getting used to pain' or 'being expected to live with pain'. Such attitudes and misconceptions are held by staff and older people themselves, and are also present within any care setting. Education of staff, relatives and older people themselves is a crucial part of effective pain management.

Multimodal management

The key to managing pain in older adults, regardless of age, is to adopt a multimodal approach rather than using one strategy. This may include pharmacological approaches, but it is far more appropriate to use lower doses of drugs along with adjuvant strategies such as relaxation, TENS, massage or similar. (These approaches are discussed in separate chapters.) Standards and protocols should be in place which can be used to monitor both individual and institutional outcomes.

All of these considerations are important, but the key to effective pain management within any setting or with any age group is education. Improving health-care staff's understanding will enable them to provide a creative approach to pain assessment and management that will be more successful. It is important to remember that pain management is a basic human right for everyone regardless of age, gender or any other factor that may influence pain perception. Therefore, any management strategy should be tailored to the individual needs of the patient, regardless of their age or clinical setting.

Conclusion

'Pain is the most frequent cause of suffering and disability that seriously impairs the quality of life for millions of people throughout the world' (Bonica and Loeser, 2001, p. 3). Numerous studies in various patient groups in both acute and other care settings show that patients often experience severe pain (Ross and Crook, 1998; Morrison and Siu, 2000; Svensson, Sjostrum and Haljamae, 2001). In clinical practice the communication of pain takes place within the context of an everyday dialogue between the patient and the nurse. Both older patients and health-care professionals believe that verbal communication is the most common way to express the pain experience (Blomqvist and Hallberg, 2001). Health-care professionals must therefore listen to what the older people in the care are saying, and respond accordingly.

References

Abbey, J., Piler, N. and DeBellis, A. *et al.* (2004) The Abbey Pain Scale: a 1-minute numerical indicator for people with end stage dementia. *International Journal of Palliative Nursing,* **10**(1), 6–13.

Adams, E.R. and McGuire, F.A. (1986) Is laughter the best medicine? A study of the effects of humor on perceived pain and affect. *Activities, Adaptation and Aging,* **8**, 157–75.

Agency for Healthcare Policy and Research (1992) Acute Pain Management Guideline Panel. *Acute Pain Management: Operative and Medical Procedures or Trauma. Clinical Practice Guideline.* AHCPR pub. No. 92–0032. Department of Health and Human Services. Public Health Service. Agency for Health Care Policy and Research, Rockville, MD.

Allcock, N., McGarry, J. and Elkan, R. (2002) Management of pain in older people within a care home: a preliminary study. *Health and Social Care in the Community,* **10**(6), 464–71.

American Geriatric Society (1998) Panel on chronic pain in older persons. The management of pain in older persons. *Journal of the American Geriatrics Society,* **46**, 635–51.

Anderson, G., Vestergaard, K., Ingeman-Nielsen, M. and Jenson, T.S. (1995) Incidence of post-stroke pain. *Pain,* **61**, 187–93.

Andersson, H.I., Ejertsson, G., Leden, I. and Rosenberg, C. (1993) Chronic pain in geographically defined general population: studies of difference in age, gender, social class and pain localization. *Clinical Journal of Pain,* **9**, 174–82.

Baltes, P.B. (1991) The many faces of human aging: toward a psychological culture of old age. *Psychological Medicine,* **21**, 837–54.

Barrowclough, C., King, P., Colville, J., Eve, R., Burns, A. and Tarrier, N. (2001) A randomised trial of the effectiveness of cognitive-behavioural therapy and supportive counselling for anxiety symptoms in older adults. *Journal of Consulting and Clinical Psychology,* **69**(5), 756–62.

Bayer, M., Bresloff, L. and Curley, D. (1986) The enhancement project: a program to improve the quality of residents' lives. *Geriatric Nursing,* **7**(4), 192–5.

Bender, J.S. (1989) Approach to the acute abdomen. *Medical Clinics of North America,* **73**, 1413–22.

Bengston, V.L., Reedy, M.N. and Gordon, C. (1985). Aging and self-conceptions: personality processes and social contexts. In J.E. Birren and K.W. Schaie (Eds.) *Handbook of the Psychology of Aging.* Van Nostrand Reinhold, New York, pp. 544–93.

Benrud-Larson, L.M. and Wegener, S.T. (2000) Chronic pain in neuro-rehabilitation populations: prevalence, severity and impact. *NeuroRehabilitation*, **14**, 127–37.

Bergh, I., Jakobsson, E., Sjostrum, B. and Steen, B. (2005) Ways of talking about experiences of pain among older patients following orthopaedic surgery. *Journal of Advanced Nursing*, **52**(4), 351–61.

Blomqvist, K. and Edberg, A. (2002) Living with persistent pain: experiences of older people receiving home care. *Journal of Advanced Nursing*, **40**(3), 297–306.

Blomqvist, K. and Hallberg, I.R. (2001) Recognizing pain in older adults living in sheltered accommodation: the views of nurses and older adults. *International Journal of Nursing Studies*, **38**(3), 305–18.

Bonica, J. and Loeser, J.D. (2001) History of pain concepts and therapies, in *J Bonica's the Management of Pain* (eds J.D. Loeser, S.H. Butler, C.R. Chapman and D.C. Turk), pp. 3–16. Lippincott Williams & Wilkins, Philadelphia.

Brockopp, D., Warden, S. and Colclough, G. *et al.* (1996) Elderly people's knowledge of and attitudes to pain management. *British Journal of Nursing*, **5**, 556–62.

Chapiro, S.L. (2001) The DOLOPLUS© 2 scale – evaluating pain in the elderly. *European Journal of Palliative Care*, **8**(5), 191–4.

Cleeland, C.S., Gonin, R., Hatfield, A.K., Edmonson, J.H., Blum, R.H., Stewart, J.A. and Pandya, K. (1994) Pain and its treatment in outpatients with metastatic breast cancer. *New England Journal of Medicine*, **330**, 592–6.

Closs, S.J. (1996) Pain and elderly patients: a survey of nurses' knowledge and experiences. *Journal of Advanced Nursing*, **23**(2), 237–42.

Closs, S.J., Barr, B., Briggs, M., Cash, K. and Seers, K. (2004) A comparison of five pain assessment scales for nursing home resident with varying degrees of cognitive impairment. *Journal of Pain and Symptom Management*, **27**(3), 196–205.

Cook, A.J. and Thomas, M.R. (1994). Pain and the use of health services among the elderly. *Journal of Aging and Health*, **6**, 155–72.

Corran, T.M., Helme, R.D. and Gibson, S.J. (2001) Multidisciplinary assessment and treatment of pain in older persons. *Topics in Geriatric Rehabilitation*, **16**(3), 1–11.

Cowan, D.T., Roberts, J.D., Fitzpatrick, J.M. and White, A.E. (2003) The need for effective assessment and management of pain among older people in care homes. *Reviews in Clinical Gerontology*, **13**, 335–41.

Davis, R.W. (1993) Phantom sensation, phantom pain and stump pain. *Archives of Physical Medicine and Rehabilitation*, **74**, 79–91.

Department of Health (2001) *National Service Framework for Older People*. The Stationery Office, London.

Elliott, A.M., Smith, B.H. and Penny, K.I. (1999) The epidemiology of chronic pain in the community. *The Lancet*, **354**(9186), 1248–52.

Erikson, E.H., Erikson, J.M. and Kivnick, H.Q. (1986) *Vital Involvement in Old Age: The Experience of Old Age in Our Time*, Norton, New York.

Ferrell, B.A. (1993) Pain, in *Ambulatory Geriatric Care* (eds T.T. Yoshikawa, E.L. Cobbs, and K. Brummel-Smith), pp. 382–90. Mosby, St Louis.

Ferrell, B.R. (1991) Pain management in elderly people. *Journal of American Geriatrics Society*, **39**, 64–73.

Ferrell, B.R. (1996) Non-drug interventions, in *Pain in the Elderly* (eds B.R. Ferrell and B.A. Ferrell), pp. 35–44. IASP Press, Seattle.

Ferrell, B.R. and Ferrell, B.A. (1996) *Pain in the Elderly*. International Association for the Study of Pain: Task Force Report. IASP Press, Seattle.

Ferrell, B.R., Ferrell, B.R. and Osterwell, D. (1990) Pain in the nursing home. *Journal of the American Geriatric Society*, **38**, 409–14.

Flor, T., Fydric, T. and Turk, D.C. (1992) Efficacy of multidisciplinary pain treatment centres: a meta-analytic review. *Pain*, **49**, 221–30.

Fordyce, W.E. (1976) *Behavioural Methods for Chronic Pain and Illness*. Mosby, St Louis.

Fox, P.L., Raina, P. and Jadad, A.R. (1999) Prevalence and treatment of pain in older adults in nursing homes and other long term care institutions: a systematic review. *Canadian Medical Association Journal*, **160**, 329–33.

Gagliese, L., Katz, J. and Melzack, R. (1999) Pain in the elderly. In R. Meizack and P.D. Wall (Eds.) *Textbook of Pain*. Churchill Livingston, Edinburgh, pp. 991–1006.

Gibson, S. (2002) *Pain in Older Persons*. Presentation at the World Pain Congress. IASP, San Diego.

Harkins, S.W., Price, D.D. and Braith, J. (1989) Effects of extraversion and neuroticism on experimental pain, clinical pain, and illness behavior. *Pain*, **36**, 209–18.

Herr, K. (2002) Chronic pain in the older patient: management strategies. *Journal of Gerontological Nursing*, **28**(2), 28–34.

Herr, K.A. and Mobily, P.R. (1991) Complexities of pain assessment in the elderly: clinical consideration. *Journal of Gerontological Nursing*, **17**, 12–19.

Hicks, T.J. (2000) Ethical implications of pain management in a nursing home: a discussion. *Nursing Ethics*, **7**(5), 392–8.

Hill, C.A. (1999) Phantom limb pain: a review of the literature on attributes and potential mechanisms. *Journal of Pain and Symptom Management*, **17**, 125–42.

Horgas, A.L. (2003) Pain management in elderly adults. *Journal of Infusion Nursing*, **26**(3), 161–5.

Hurley, A.C., Volicer, P.A. and Hanrahan, P.A. *et al.* (1992) Assessment of discomfort in advanced Alzheimer patients. *Research in Nursing and Health*, **15**, 369–77.

Kahana, B., Kahana, E., Namazi, K., Kercher, K. and Strange, K. (1997) The role of pain in the cascade from chronic illness to social disability and psychosocial distress in later life, in *Handbook of Pain and Aging* (eds D.I. Mostofsky and J. Lomranz), pp. 185–206. Academic Press, New York.

Kane, R.L., Ouslander, J.G. and Abrass, I.B. (1989) *Essentials of Clinical Geriatrics*, 2nd edn. McGraw-Hill, New York.

Keefe, F. and Williams, D.A. (1990). A comparison of coping strategies in chronic pain patients in different age groups. *Journal of Gerontology: Psychological Sciences*, **45**, 161–5.

Lovheim, H., Sandman, P.O., Kallin, K., Karlson, S. and Gustafson, Y. (2006) Poor awareness of analgesic treatment jeopardizes adequate pain control in the care of older people. *Age and Aging*, **35**(3), 257–61.

Lumme-Sandt, K., Hervonen, A. and Jylla, M. (2000) Interpretive repertoires of medication among the oldest-old. *Social Science and Medicine*, **50**, **12**, 1843–50.

McCaffery, M. and Pasero, C. (1995) Selected barriers to pain management in the elderly, in *Pain in the Elderly* (eds B.R. Ferrell and B.A. Ferrell), IASP Press, Seattle.

Melding, P.S. (1991) Is there such a thing as geriatric pain? Guest editorial. *Pain*, **46**, 119–21.

Melzack, R. and Wall, P. (1990) *The Challenge of Pain*. Penguin, London.

Middaugh, S.J., Woods, S.E., Kee, W.G., Harden, R.N. and Peters, J.R. (1991) Biofeedback assisted relaxation training for the aging chronic pain patient. *Biofeedback and Self-regulation*, **16**, 361–77.

Miller, C. and LeLieuvre, R.B. (1982) A method to reduce chronic pain in elderly nursing home residents. *The Gerontologist*, **22**, 314–17.

Mobiliy, P.R., Herr, K.A., Clark, M.K. and Wallace, R.B. (1994) An epidemiologic analysis of pain in the elderly: the Iowa 65+ Rural Health Study. *Journal of Aging and Health*, **6**, 139–54.

Morgan, J.P. (1985) American opiophobia: customary underutilization of opioid analgesics. *Advances in Alcohol and Substance Abuse*, 5(1–2), 163–73.

Morrison, R.S. and Siu, A.L. (2000) A comparison of pain and its treatment in advanced dementia and cognitively intact patients with hip fracture. *Journal of Pain Symptom Management*, **19**(4), 240–8.

Moye, J. and Hanlon, S. (1996) Relaxation training for nursing home patients: suggestions for simplifying and individualizing treatment. *Clinical Gerontologist*, **16**(3), 37–48.

Popp, B. and Portenoy, R.K. (1996) Management of chronic pain in the elderly: pharmacology of opioids and other analgesic drugs, in *Pain in the Elderly* (eds B.A. Ferrell and B.R. Ferrell), pp. 21–34. IASP Press, Seattle.

Reid, M.C., Otis, J., Barry, L.C. and Kerns, R.D. (2003) Cognitive- behavioural therapy for chronic low back pain in older persons: a preliminary study. *Pain Medicine*, **4**, 233–0.3.

Riley, J.L., Wade, J.B., Robinson, M.E. and Price, D.D. (2000) The stages of pain processing across the adult lifespan. *The Journal of Pain*, **1**, 162–70.

Roberto, K.A. and Gold, D.T. (2001) *Chronic Pain in Later Life: A Selectively Annotated Bibliography*. Greenwood Press, Westport, CT.

Ross, M.M. and Crook, J. (1998) Elderly recipients of nursing home services: pain, disability and functional competence. *Journal of Advanced Nursing*, **27**(6), 1117–26.

Schumacher, K.L., West, C., Dodd, M., Paul, S.M., Tripathy, D., Koo, P. and Miaskowski, C.A. (2002) Pain management autobiographies and reluctance to use opioids for cancer pain management. *Cancer Nursing*, **25**(2), 125–33.

Secker, D.L., Kazantzis, N. and Pachana, N.A. (2004) Cognitive-behavioural therapy for older adults: practical guidelines for adapting therapy structure. *Journal of Rational Emotive and Cognitive-Behavioural Therapy*, **22**(2), 93–109.

Senstaken, E.A. and King, S.A. (1993) The problems of pain and its detection among geriatric nursing home residents. *Journal of the American Geriatrics Society*, **41**, 541–4.5.

Shapiro, R.S. (1994) Liability issues in the management of pain. *Journal of Pain and Symptom Management*, **9**(3), 146–52.

Simons, W. and Malabar, R. (1995) Assessing pain in elderly patients who cannot respond verbally. *Journal of Advanced Nursing*, **22**, 663–9.

Sorkin, B.A., Rudy, T.E., Hanlon, R.B., Turk, D.C. and Steig, R.L. (1990) Chronic pain in old and young patients: differences appear less important than similarities. *Journal of Gerontology: Psychological Sciences*, **45**, 64–8.

Stuck, A.E., Siu, A.L., Wieland, A.D., Adams, J. and Rubenstein, L.Z. (1993) Comprehensive geriatric assessment: a meta-analysis of controlled trials. *Lancet*, **342**, 1032–6.

Svensson, I., Sjostrum, B. and Haljamae, H. (2001) Influence of expectations and actual pain experiences on satisfaction with post-operative pain management. *European Journal of Pain*, **5**(2), 125–33.

Turk, D.C., Meichenbaum, D. and Genest, M. (1983) *Pain and Behavioural Medicine: A Cognitive Behavioural Perspective*. Guilford Press, New York.

Valkenburg, H.A. (1988) Epidemiologic considerations of the geriatric population. *Gerontology*, **34**(Suppl. 1), 2–10.

Walker, J.M., Akinsanya, J.A., David, B.D. and Marcer, D.M. (1990) The management of elderly patients in pain in the community: study and recommendations. *Journal of Pain and Symptom Management*, **10**, 204–31.

Won, A.B., Lapane, K.L. and Vallow, S. et al. (2004) Persistent nonmalignant pain and analgesic prescribing patterns in elderly nursing home residents. *Journal of the American Geriatric Society*, **52**(6), 867–74.

World Health Organization (1990) *Cancer Pain Relief and Palliative Care*. WHO, Geneva.

Yates, P. and Fentiman, B. (1995) Pain: the views of elderly people living in long-term residential care settings. *Journal of Advanced Nursing*, **21**(4), 667–74.

Yonan, C.A. and Wegener, S.T. (2003) Assessment and management of pain in the older adult. *Rehabilitation Psychology*, **48**(1), 4–13.

Management of a pain by pharmacological intervention in older adults

9

Rachel Drago

The aims of this chapter are to explore common concepts general to pharmacology and to apply them to the effects that age has on the physiological functioning of the human body.

- What is pharmacology?
- Principles of pharmacokinetics, pharmacodynamics, bioavailability.
- Effects of senescence upon the body, changes in body systems with ageing.
- Senescence and drugs; clinical considerations.

Principles of pharmacology

Pharmacology is the study of the interaction between chemicals and the human body. It can be broken down into two distinct disciplines: the study of the body systems on the chemical and the study of the effects of the chemical upon the body systems. It is important to remember that all drugs have both positive and negative effects on the body. The negative consequences are called **adverse reactions** or **side effects**. It is vital to weigh up the risks of a drug versus the benefits when embarking upon drug therapy.

Pharmacokinetics – what the body does to the drug

Pharmacokinetics is the study of the time course of the drug through the body from the site of administration to the elimination of the drug from the body. It generally entails four principles: absorption, distribution, biotransformation and elimination.

Absorption

Absorption from the site of administration involves the drug crossing epithelial membranes – the lipid bilayer of cell membranes – and it is determined by factors such as the fat (lipid) solubility of the drug, its size and molecular weight, and its concentration gradient across the membrane. Very small, highly fat-soluble drugs will pass through epithelial and cell membranes more quickly than large, complex, highly water-soluble drugs.

The rate and extent of drug absorption from the site of administration determine its **bioavailability**. This is the proportion of the dose given which reaches the systemic circulation unaltered. For 100% bioavailability, all of the drug must reach the systemic circulation; this can be achieved with certainty only by intravenous administration. Orally administered drugs often have a reduced bioavailability due to the action of gut acids and digestive and biotransformation enzymes on the drug as it passes through the gut lining, into the hepatic portal system and then on through the liver. This is termed the **first pass effect**. As the drug passes through the liver, the enzymes there remove a proportion of the active drug from the circulation, thereby reducing the overall amount of drug that reaches the systemic circulation. This goes some way to explaining why oral doses tend in general to be some what larger than their injected formulations.

Learning point

Revise the anatomy of the blood flow from the gut to the liver and check out your knowledge of the hepatic portal system.

Distribution

A drug is distributed around the body from the site of absorption by dissolving in the plasma, or by attaching to plasma proteins or haemoglobin or via carrier molecules. Once in the systemic circulation the drug is only active if unbound from plasma proteins.

Drug delivery to all tissues is dependent upon how effective the pump is and how patent the tubing is through which it passes – in other words, the condition of the circulation. A poor pump and blocked tubing prevent the distribution of a drug to the body. Hence, people with cardiac failure and atherosclerosis often suffer from the consequences of poor distribution to under-perfused tissues. An example is the peripheral hypoxia and venous hypertension which manifest with peripheral ulcers that become colonized with bacteria, leading to chronic infection. The poor delivery system precludes an adequate delivery of systemic antibiotics and hence the ulcer remains chronically colonized and infected.

Biotransformation

Sometimes referred to as **metabolism**, this occurs predominately in the liver but also in the lining of the small intestine, lungs and kidneys. The process of 'breaking down' exogenous drugs and endogenous compounds such as steroid hormones is carried out by a family of intracellular enzymes known as cytochrome P450 (cyp450). Within the liver other isoenzymes are responsible for the breakdown of specific chemicals: an example is alcohol dehydrogenase, an enzyme which catalyses the breakdown of alcohol. Other enzymes bind (conjugate) drugs to proteins and sulfates to produce large, water-soluble molecules.

Cyp450 enzymes are effective in the reduction, hydrolysis or oxidation of drugs to make them less active and less effective; they render the drug harmless and make it water-soluble so that it can be removed from the body via the water-based waste systems. Cyp450 enzymes can be inhibited by concomitant ingestion of grapefruit juice or cranberry juice. These fruit juices, in small quantities, inhibit the cyp450 found in the gut lining, thus increasing the quantity of drug which enters the hepatic portal circulation. Larger quantities of grapefruit juice will inhibit the cyp450 found in the liver. The end effect is to increase the bioavailability of a given drug. In the case of dose-sensitive drugs such as warfarin a marked change in the blood coagulability and decrease in clotting (INR) can be noted after just one small glass of grapefruit juice (Baily et al., 1998).

As well as being inhibited, the action and quantity of cyp450 enzymes can also be enhanced. Direct induction of the liver enzymes results in the rapid biotransformation of a given drug, so that the bioavailability falls with oral administration and the overall therapeutic duration of action is reduced. With a dose-sensitive drugs such as the oral contraceptive pill, concomitant use of St Johns wort inevitably results in therapeutic failure as the contraceptive is rapidly rendered ineffective by the induced cyp450 system.

It is this mechanism of cyp450 induction and inhibition that forms the major cause of drug interactions when a patient is taking more than one pharmaceutical therapy. Enzyme induction is also a considerable cause of tolerance to a number of addictive drugs, such as benzodiazepines, barbiturates and alcohol. However, it is important to point out that this is not the cause of opiate tolerance, which is brought about by the down-regulation of opiate receptors in the central nervous system, and not through pharmacokinetic changes to the liver enzymes.

As mentioned earlier, other enzymes which do not form part of the cyp450 system are also present in liver cells. Their function is to bind the drug molecule to proteins and sulfates. Again the aim is to make the drug molecule ineffective and more water soluble.

Biotransformation can be divided into those reactions that are carried out by cyp450 and those that require enzymes to bind the drug molecule with another substance:

- **Phase 1 biotransformation** is the biological changing of a drug by the cyp450 system
- **Phase 2 biotransformation** is the conjugation of drugs by other liver enzymes

Some drugs are extensively biotransformed by phase 1 reactions, others by phase 2 and some by both. Other drugs are eliminated without biotransformation and leave the body in the same form they entered it. Health-care practitioners should study the product literature published by the drug manufacturers to better understand which reaction (if any) is responsible for the breakdown of a particular drug.

For most drugs, given at the correct dose and time interval, biotransformation processes do indeed result in a less active/reactive and more easily eliminated substance. There are exceptions, in which a drug can be made more reactive and potentially more poisonous by the natural biotransformation processes: an example is paracetamol. In prescribed doses a tiny proportion of paracetamol is metabolized by the cyp450 system into a highly hepatotoxic metabolite. This metabolite is then conjugated with glutathionine to form a larger and harmless end product which can be eliminated from the body. However, if paracetamol is consumed in greater doses than recommended, or with other substances, such as alcohol, which also depend on glutathionine for conjugation, then the toxic paracetamol metabolite can accumulate and damage liver cells irreversibly.

Another example is the conjugation reaction of morphine with glucuronide to produce morphine-6-glucuronide, which is a highly effective opiate receptor agonist and remains active within the central nervous system until eliminated by the kidney(Osborne et al., 1992).

Hepatic insufficiency results in the slow biotransformation of drugs by the cyp450 and conjugation enzymes, leading to potential drug toxicity. The British National Formulary advises very clearly about drug doses and time intervals, and which drugs to avoid, in case of hepatic impairment.

Revise the structure and functions of the liver.

Elimination

The drug or metabolite (the end product of the biotransformation processes) is eliminated from the body predominately through the kidneys, carried in the urine, but also in the water vapour in the breath, in the sweat, in the bile and (for lactating women) secreted in the breast milk. Elimination of most drugs is dependent upon the health of the kidneys, including renal blood flow and glomerular filtration rate (GFR). Normal GFR is 100 ml/min for each 1.73 m^2 of body surface area (a 'standard' body size). A GFR of less than 100 indicates some degree of renal insufficiency and can result in the build-up of drug metabolites within the plasma, which in turn can lead to drug toxicity, adverse reactions and even death. In the case of renal insufficiency drug dosages and time intervals need to be carefully considered to prevent this. Again, the BNF advises very carefully on prescribing in renal insufficiency.

Revise the structure and function of the renal system, especially the glomerular filtration, absorption and secretion processes of urine formation.

Figure 9.1 shows the rapid increase in systemic plasma concentration as the drug is absorbed from the gut, passing through the gut lining, entering the

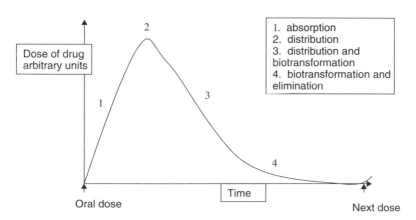

1. absorption
2. distribution
3. distribution and biotransformation
4. biotransformation and elimination

Figure 9.1 The pharmacokinetics of an oral dose of a drug over time

hepatic portal system, through the liver and into the systemic circulation, where it is distributed throughout the body. The plasma concentration drops as the drug is fully distributed and begins to be biotransformed and finally eliminated. If a further dose is not forthcoming, the drug level will finally fall to zero. The kinetic of an intravenous bolus will not demonstrate the absorption phase, as the drug is administered directly to the systemic circulation; hence the drug begins with a peak plasma level that gradually falls as the drug is distributed, biotransformed and eliminated.

Pharmacodynamics – what the drug does to the body, how the drug alters physiological function

Drugs and chemicals have been used as a therapy for the treatment of pathological or age-related changes since ancient times. The father of pharmacology, Paracelsus, said that the only difference between a therapy and poison is the dose at which it is given. All drugs produce side effects and have the propensity for interactions and adverse reactions.

Drugs bring about both their therapeutic and their adverse effects by acting on receptors, ion channels, enzymes or carrier molecules, or by direct chemical reaction.

Receptors

On cell membranes and within the cytoplasm there are receptors with a specific affinity for a particular neurotransmitter or hormone. A receptor will only bind with the specific hormone or neurotransmitter that fits it, just as a key will only open a particular lock. For example, an opiate receptor only has affinity for opiate neurotransmitters or opiate-like drugs and will not respond to other hormones or neurotransmitters. This forms the basis of the lock-and-key theory of receptor binding (Figure 9.2).

Drugs are developed to stimulate or block receptors, for example opiate analgesics stimulate opiate receptors found within the central nervous system. The opiate receptors are stimulated with morphine which will decrease the sensitivity of the transmission neurons to pain-producing stimuli and neurotransmitters such as substance P and glutamate, thus ameliorating the perception of pain. Equally you can intensify the pain experience by blocking the opiate receptors with naloxone.

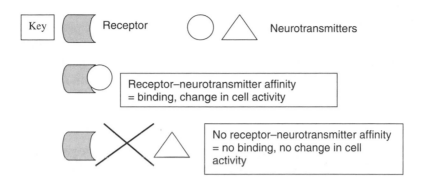

Figure 9.2 Simplified lock and key mechanism

Table 9.1 Receptors and agonist/antagonist drugs

Receptor	Agonist	Antagonist
Adrenoreceptors	Noradrenalin, salbutamol	Propranolol, atenolol
Cholinergic	Acetylcholine, pilocarpine	Atropine, hyoscine
Serotonin	Sumatriptan (receptor subtype1)	Ondansetron (receptor subtype 3)
	Metoclopramide (receptor subtype 4)	Dihydroerogotamine (receptor subtype2)
Opioid	Morphine	Naloxone

Learning points

- A drug which shows affinity for a receptor and activates that receptor is called an **agonist**.
- A drug which shows affinity for a receptor but prevents its activation is called an **antagonist**

Morphine is an opiate receptor agonist.
Naloxone is an opiate receptor antagonist (Table 9.1)

Ion channels

Ion channels are found with in the cell membranes of all cells. Ion channels are of particular importance in excitable cells. Excitable cells are those cells which are able to generate electrical charges, such as nerve cells and muscle cells. It is the opening or closing ion channels that alters the intracellular and extracellular balance of ions across the cell membrane.

Learning point

Ions are charged particles, such as sodium ions (Na^+), potassium ions (K^+), chloride ions (Cl^-), calcium ions (Ca^{2+}), magnesium ions (Mg^{2+}).

Changing ion balance across excitable cell membranes will affect the conductivity of nerves and the ability of all types of muscle tissue to contract and relax. Therefore many drugs which are **ion channel blockers** make very good muscle relaxants and local anaesthetics. Calcium channel blockers such as nifedipine cause relaxation of vascular and cardiac smooth muscle by stopping the inward flow of calcium into smooth muscle cells, thus reducing the force of contraction, decreasing vascular resistance and producing a reduction in blood pressure.

Local anaesthetics such as lignocaine and xylocaine block the inward current of sodium ions into the sensory nerve endings, thus preventing the nerve from depolarizing and generating the microelectrical charge which causes the action potential (nerve impulse). As the nerve is unable to produce an action potential, the afferent nerves sending sensory information to the central nervous system stop firing and a total lack of sensation results. How long this lasts depends on the half-life of the drug and whether it is administered by bolus injection or by infusion, as with epidural anaesthesia in childbirth and postoperative analgesia.

Enzyme cascades

Both intracellular and extracellular enzyme cascades regulate and maintain **homeostasis**.

Leaning point

Homeostasis is the maintenance of a constant and yet dynamic internal environment regardless of the changes in the external environment.

Many biochemical and physiological processes are determined by enzyme reactions (see Chapter 1). The experience of dull, chronic, throbbing pain is a result of tissue damage and tissue enzymes producing pain-potentiating chemicals such as prostaglandins, bradykinin, serotonin and leukotrienes, which are sometimes known as local hormones. These chemicals actively increase the sensitivity of the pain fibres and promote the sensation of pain within the central nervous system; this is central sensitization (see Chapter 1). Blocking the enzymes responsible for the production of the inflammatory and pain-promoting chemicals can reduce the individual's experience of pain. Aspirin and other non-steroidal anti-inflammatory drugs (NSAIDs) work like this. They inhibit the action of the enzyme cyclooxygenase (COX) on arachidonic acid, and prevent the conversion of arachidonate into local hormones (Table 9.2).

Learning point

The use of aspirin and other NSAIDs results in the inhibition of all forms of COX. COX is responsible for the formation of homeostatic gastric and renal protective prostaglandins which regulate the diameter of the vessels supplying the stomach lining and kidney with oxygen-rich blood. These prostaglandins ensure that the vessels remain relaxed and hence the flow of blood and oxygen is plentiful. When you take aspirin all prostaglandin formation stops, the gut vessels constrict, resistance to blood flow increases and blood volume to the stomach lining and kidney falls, leading to a potentially harmful tissue hypoxia. Hypoxia results in ischaemia, with the consequence of stomach ulceration and glomerular damage. The speed with which this occurs varies from individual to individual.

Carrier molecules

These exist within the cell membranes and epithelia specifically for the transport of large substances which cannot pass through the membrane passively, or for moving chemicals against the diffusion gradient. **Proton pump inhibitors** (PPIs) are good examples of carrier molecule inhibitors. These drugs prevent the movement of hydrogen ions into the gastric secretions, thus reducing the acidity (raising the pH) of the gastric juices. The use of concomitant PPIs with NSAIDs in patients with chronic inflammatory pain conditions has been shown to ameliorate the gastric ulceration associated with the use of NSAIDs.

Table 9.2 Examples of enzymes, the drugs that inhibit them and their therapeutic effects

Enzyme	Inhibiting drug	Therapeutic effect
Angiotensin converting enzyme	Captopril	Reducs blood pressure
Cyclooxygenases 1, 2 and 3	Aspirin	Anti-inflammatory, analgesic
Phospholipase	Corticosteroids	Anti-inflammatory
Acetylcholinesterase	Organophosphates	Insecticides
Monoamine oxidase A	Iproniazide	Antidepressant
Monoamine oxidase B	Selegiline	Antidepressant
HMG-CoA reductase	Simvastatin	Reduces cholesterol
Xanthine oxidase	Allopurinol	Prevents gout
DNA polymerase	Cytarabine	Cytotoxic
Clotting cascade	Heparin	Anticoagulant
DNA synthesis	Azathiaprine	Disease-modifying drugs

Direct chemical reaction

One type of drug that works by direct chemical reaction is antacids, which use an alkali or basic chemical, such as sodium bicarbonate, to neutralize the acidic gastric juices to produce a brief but effective respite from heartburn.

Leaning point

By understanding the principles by which pharmacology is defined one can see how drugs work, why they have to be given by specific administration routes over specific time intervals, and why care must be taken in cases of hepatic and renal insufficiency.

- Try to apply this knowledge to your practice. Think about the drugs you administer regularly. Are there any important considerations about route of administration? For example, penicillin G can only be given intravenously as it is remarkably water soluble and has limited lipid solubility, so it would never cross the gut lining if given by the oral route.

Summary

- **Pharmacokinetics:** What the body does to the drug; the time course of the drug through the body, comprising of absorption, distribution, biotransformation and elimination. It also involves the principle of bioavailability, the percentage of the drug given which reaches the system circulation unaltered.

- **Pharmacodynamics:** What the drug does to the body either by acting on receptors, ion channels, enzyme cascades or carrier molecules, or by direct chemical reaction. Ultimately the functioning of the body is changed to produce a desired effect and all too often an undesired or side effect. All drugs have side effects; the practitioner must weight up the risk of side effects versus the benefit of the drugs and plan to met these side effects, preferably before they occur. For example: anticipating and preventing the inevitable side effect of constipation with opiate use by the co-prescribing of laxatives. The same could be said for preventing nausea and vomiting, which is experienced by half the patients who are prescribed opiate analgesia.

- **Biotransformation:** The biological alteration of drugs and hormones into inactive water-soluble excretable molecules. Biotransformation of drugs can be increased by inducing liver enzymes, resulting in therapy failure.

- Inhibiting liver enzymes will result in **drug toxicity** as the drug remains in the circulation in its active much longer.

- **Kidney failure** will result in the retention of active drugs and the metabolites. In case of active metabolites such as morphine-6-glucuronide, a sustained effect from the morphine will be seen.

Normal physiological changes in older adults

With some minor exceptions, drugs tend to produce greater and more prolonged effects with increasing age. This is largely due to the changes in the physiological responsiveness of the older human body (Mangoni and Jackson, 2003). Just as we insist that children are not adults in miniature and that their physiology is specific to their age group, the same principle should be applied to older adults. People of advanced years are not a young adults in a more mature shell! Older people have distinct physiological features that are due entirely to age and not to pathological processes. However, we have medicalized ageing and used a pathology-based approach to old age which has manifested itself in the attempted treatment of many natural occurrences of senescence.

In a society where youth is idolized and ageing shunned, we have come to believe that all of the changes we encounter in our body as we grow older can be treated, tucked and pinned to maintain our youthful exuberance, if not necessarily the quality of life. But, as mentioned earlier in this chapter, all drugs are poisons and it is simply the dose at which the drug is given which distinguishes poisoning from therapy. All drugs have side effects and these side effects are the culprit in a number of iatrogenic diseases and the polypharmacy often seen in older patients. Many highly regarded practitioners in the care of older adults suggest that we should not be putting 'years into life' but 'life into the years'. Pain is a major issue which should be assessed effectively and treated using a multidimensional approach, not just pharmacologically.

Body composition, water, muscle and fat volumes change naturally with age, as do the cardiovascular, hepatic, renal and integumentary systems. At a microscopic level there is evidence to suggest that sensory neurons decrease in number and sensitivity; there are alterations to receptor numbers, affinity and sensitivity. These changes slow reflexes, reduce muscle strength and alter the delicate homeostatic mechanisms which maintain the internal environment of the body at optimal levels. In health these changes do not pose a major problem to the individual, but in disease or ill-health requiring pharmacological intervention these changes must be included in the equation when considering treatment, administration route, doses and time interval.

Learning point

Drug information booklets are usually based on the assessment of pharmacokinetic profile of a drug in young male healthy subjects, and trials are not carried out in older subjects for obvious ethical reasons.

Integumentary and musculoskeletal changes

With increasing age the proportion of muscle to fat changes. Fast twitch muscle fibres in the large muscles of the quadriceps, gluteus and biceps decline in number, reducing reaction speed and strength. The overall muscle mass falls (Grimby and Saltin, 1983) and although there is no obvious increase in fat levels, the ratio of lean active, metabolic tissue to fat decreases, thus lowering the individual's overall metabolic rate. A lower muscle mass will also decrease the 24-hour output of creatinine (a by-product of muscle contraction which is totally cleared by the kidneys; Martini, 1998).

Skin loses elasticity as a result of collagen loss and elastin degradation. The skin wrinkles and subcutaneous fat thins (Martini, 1998). Fat is deposited deeper into the body cavities. Vessels in the skin are also reduced in number and become less reactive to temperature changes; hence, overall skin blood flow is less.

Absorption via the injection and transdermal drug administration routes can be reduced or prolonged in the older adult. Empirical evidence to support this is very difficult to find, but when using these routes for the first time in older patients you should pay particular attention to speed of onset and duration of action to ascertain absorption from these routes.

There is anecdotal evidence of potential drug bolus dosing arising from subcutaneous administration routes in cold older patients. The transdermal patches used were designed to release a set dose per hour of a drug into the subcutaneous fat. Under normal circumstances the drug is then absorbed into the bloodstream and distributed around the body. However, if the blood flow to the skin is reduced temporarily because of cold, shock or pathological processes, the patch will still release the set dose hourly, so it accumulates in the subcutaneous tissue only to be absorbed rapidly into the blood when tissue perfusion increases. This may be anecdotal, and the empirical evidence too limited to suggest a nationwide problem, but nevertheless it is essential that we should assess any potential accumulation of drugs in our older patients. Accumulation of night sedation, opiates or even sedating antihistamines provides the patients with a potential minefield of problems, ranging from decreased mental alertness and confusion to difficulty in mobilizing and incontinence.

The issue also arises when administering drugs by the intramuscular route. Inactive patients have reduced muscle perfusion, which in turn reduces rate of absorption and distribution.

Oral administration is a very haphazard method of administration in all humans and is subject to a great deal of individual variability, even more so in older adults, as a result of changes in gut pH. Especially in the stomach acidity levels fall with age, as does gut motility and effective surface area for absorption. Drug side effects have a much greater impact on the bowel in older adults; both constipation and diarrhoea seem to present more commonly. Again this evidence is anecdotal, as empirical data are currently lacking.

Cardiovascular changes

In healthy older adults cardiovascular changes do not present a problem, but pathological changes to the heart and vessels such as ventricular failure and hardening of the arteries will impact on the distribution of drugs. A degree of realism has to be used when administering drugs and assessing the results. In some cases cure is not the goal; amelioration of symptoms may be the desired end point.

Hepatic changes

Liver enzymes are reduced with advancing age, and the rate and extent of this reduction is highly variable among individuals. Nevertheless it is widely accepted that older adults have a reduced capacity for drug metabolism. Highly fat-soluble drugs such as diazepam, alcohol, opiate analgesics and anaesthetics will remain in the body for longer than the recognized half-life because of the reduced speed of biotransformation and also to the fall in basal metabolic rate in conjunction with changes in lean tissue to fat ratio.

Renal changes

Renal function, as measured by GFR, deteriorates from the age of 20 years.

Learning points

- Normal adult GFR is 100 ml/min per 1.73 m² of body surface area.
- By the age of 50 years the glomerular filtration rate has fallen by 25%.
- By the age of 75 years GFR has fallen by 50% (Ewy *et al.*, 1969)

This change in GFR is reflected in a reduced rate of renal drug elimination. Drugs with active metabolites that are eliminated through the kidneys will accumulate and have a prolonged effect in older adults. Hence it is common to see excessive sedation and dysphoria following morphine administration due both to the side effects of morphine and the accumulation of the active metabolite morphine-6-glucuronide.

Traditional tests for urea, electrolytes and creatinine levels are not a good indicator of renal function in older adults, as levels remain stable throughout adult life due to the reduction in creatinine synthesis because of a decreased muscle mass. A failure to recognize and react to the fall in kidney function despite normal creatinine levels can lead to drug toxicity in older adults. For example, digoxin is completely eliminated by the renal route in its active form and to prevent glycoside toxicity the dosage must be halved in older adults. Today medical biochemical laboratories will provide an *estimated* glomerular filtration rate (eGFR) for individual patients, based on serum creatinine, age, sex and race. However, it has only a 90% confidence interval and is not applicable to all races, and also it assumes that the creatinine level is stable and not changing. In other words 90% of patients tested will have a GFR within 30% of the estimated GFR. Nevertheless, it can provide the practitioner with a better indication of the ability of the kidney to eliminate drugs and therefore prevent possible toxicity problems.

Sensitivity changes

It is now well understood that sensitivity to drugs in older people can cause a number of problems. For instance, diazepam and related drugs cause less sedation but more confusion and memory loss than in young adults. Opiates tend to cause dysphoria rather than euphoria, and have marked constipating qualities. Also, because of the reduced speed of cardiac and spinal reflexes and the inflexibility of arteries, opiates and hypotensives will bring about a marked degree of postural hypotension in older adults. All of these changes can lead to the misdiagnosis of age-related memory problems, falls and fractures. Hence, a drug history is vital in all cases of acute confusion in older adults.

Conclusion

It may seem from this chapter that ageing holds nothing in store but gradual decline. This is not really the case, although we have taken the hardest possible line in an effort to draw practitioners' attention to older adults as a special case of need when helping them to manage their medications and analgesia. There are far too many instances of iatrogenic disease resulting from drugs and polypharmacy in older adults. Problems of accumulation and toxicity can be avoided through the recognition of and attention to age-related physiological changes. Care with administration routes, dosages and time intervals may prevent some common problems, as will patient education and support (Jackson, Mangoni and Batty, 2003).

References

Baily, D.G., Malcolm, J., Arnold, O. and Spence, J.D. (1998) Grapefruit juice–drug interations. *British Journal of Pharmacology*, **46**, 101–10.

Ewy, G.A., Kapaclia, G.G., Yeo, L., Lullin, M. and Markus, F. (1969) Digoxin metabolism in the elderly. *Circulation*, **34**, 449–53.

Grimby, G. and Saltin, B. (1983) The ageing muscle: a mini review. *Clinical Physiology*, **3**, 209–18.

Jackson, S.H.D., Mangoni, A.A. and Batty, G.M. (2003) Optimization of drug prescribing. *British Journal of Clinical Pharmacology*, **57**(3), 231–6.

Mangoni, A.A. and Jackson, S.H.D. (2003) Age related changes in pharmacokinetics and pharmacodynamics, basic principle and practical applications. *British Journal of clinical Pharmacology*, **57**(1), 6–14.

Osborne, R., Thompson, P., Joel, S., Trew, S., Patel, N. and Slevin, M. (1992) Analgesic activity of morphine-6-glucuronide. *British Journal of Clinical Pharmacology*, **34**, 130–8.

Further reading

Greenstein, B. (2004) *Trounce's Clinical Pharmacology for Nurses*, 17th edn. Churchill Livingstone, Edinburgh.

Jones, D.A., Round, J.M. (1992) *Skeletal Muscle in Health and Disease*. Manchester University Press, Manchester.

Kumar, P. and Clark, M. (2005) *Clinical Medicine*, 6th edn. Elsevier Saunders, Philadelphia.

Martini, F.H. (1998) *Fundamentals of Anatomy and Physiology*, 4th edn. International Edition, Prentice-Hall, Englewood Cliffs, NJ.

Rang, H.P., Dale, M.M., Ritter, J.M. and Moore, P.K. (2003) *Pharmacology*, 5th edn. Churchill Livingstone, Edinburgh.

Sproule, B., Hardy, B.G. and Shulman, K. (2000) Differential pharmacokinetics in elderly patients. *Drugs and Aging*, **16**, 165–77.

Walker, R. and Edwards, C. (2003) *Clinical Pharmacy and Therapeutic*, 3rd edn. Churchill Livingstone, Edinburgh.

Waller, D.G., Renwick, A.G. and Hillier, K. (2001) *Pharmacology and Therapeutics*. WB Saunders. Philadephia.

Complementary approaches

10

Pat Schofield

Introduction

The use of complementary and alternative medicine (CAM) is gaining 'grass root support, due to its intuitive appeal' (DH, 1993), despite the lack of systematic evidence and rigorous exploration of the effects of complementary therapies. Although such approaches have been criticized for their lack of empirical evidence (Howell, 1993), there appears to be evidence of a growing demand for them within the general population (Montbriand, 1993).

CAM is defined as:

> Diagnosis, treatment and/or prevention which complements mainstream medicine by contributing to a common whole, by satisfying a demand not met by orthodoxy or by diversifying the conceptual framework of medicine (Ernst *et al.* 1995, p. 506)

Although CAM therapies are often not part of mainstream health care, they are becoming increasingly popular with the general public. For example, a study by Murray and Shepherd (1988) explored the use and prevalence of complementary therapies within a group of patients registered in a South London general practice. This was a preliminary study, carried out in only two age groups (70 and 35 year olds), but it showed that a high proportion of patients used such therapies: 25/27 (92%) of the 70 year olds and 53/80 (66%) of the 35 year olds.

The therapies being used ranged from counselling, hypnosis, massage, hypnotherapy and homeopathy to fortune telling and private allergy clinics. The patients commented that the holistic nature of these CAM approaches was more acceptable to them than traditional medicine. Some even commented that the medical profession tended to group patients together according to diagnosis and on the whole they believed that the NHS was too scientific, missing the human factor.

It is usually suggested that lack of data regarding safety or efficacy prohibits the use of CAM. However, some of these therapies seem to have a longer history than some of the traditional medical techniques. In fact TENS has been reported as being used by the Romans in the form of electric eels. Ötzi, the 'Bronze Age man' discovered in 1991 frozen in the Austrian Alps, was found to have acupuncture marks. During the last decade CAM therapies have become increasingly used as an adjuvant to traditional medical techniques, and there has been a move by the Department of Health (DH) to acknowledge such approaches and recommend how some CAM methods can be incorporated into mainstream health. For example, they make recommendations for certain approaches to be used within primary care (DH, 2000)

Learning point

Access the DH (2000) document *Complementary Medicine: Information Pack for Primary Care Groups* and read what is said about their use in the community. (see DH web site at end of chapter)

There are some independent reviews of clinical trials into CAM, for example by the Australian Expert Committee on Complementary Medicines in the Health System, by the National Center for Complementary and Alternative Medicine (NCCAM), part of the US National Institutes of Health, and by the Cochrane Collaboration (see web sites at end of chapter). Nevertheless, more research is still needed for some therapies.

Why are CAM therapies so appealing?

A number of reasons have been suggested for this:

- CAM provides a holistic perspective that encompasses quality of life and recognizes the interplay between the mind, body and environment.
- The individual can become engaged in the therapy and consequently empowered to be involved in their own management.

- CAM therapies may be more acceptable than western medicine to people of different ethnic, socio-cultural and religious groups who form part of our modern multicultural society.
- Some individuals may be disempowered by highly technical medical interventions.
- Therapists may provide more 'time' and 'pleasant environments', thus enabling the development of a stronger, more trusting relationship. It has been suggested that a placebo effect can occur with physicians or therapists which can actually produce endogenous opioids (Tie Riet et al., 1998)
- CAM therapies are usually non-invasive, and as such may be perceived to be less dangerous or more appealing.

In contrast to the positive effects of CAM therapies, there are also negative factors which have been highlighted:

- Many therapies are not regulated, so individuals need to be wary of the practitioner's experience and qualifications.
- Some therapies can be quite expensive: for example, £80 for an initial consultation followed by further costs for subsequent treatments.
- Some therapies can be contraindicated, produce side effects or even prove to be potentially harmful if not applied by appropriately trained practitioners. For example, there have been reports of serious complications associated with acupuncture including pneumothorax, cardiac tamponade, infections and even death. Some aromatherapy oils can cause asthma attacks and miscarriage, and TENS can cause cardiac pacemakers to stop functioning.

What complementary therapies are available?

Some of the most widely available are:

- **Acupuncture**: Chinese medical approach that involves inserting needles into specific points on the skin.
- **Alexander technique**: A balance of the head and neck and a suppleness of the back that makes it seem long and wide, and coordination of the limbs so they seem to function from the back, thus providing a method of self-carriage.
- **Aromatherapy**: Essential oils produced from plants and flowers are used to bring about emotional and physical changes. Oils are massaged into the skin, added to bath water or evaporated using an oil burner.

- **Ayurveda**: An ancient Indian healing system that suggests that illness is cause by an imbalance of the body's vital energy forces. Combines the use of yoga, massage, acupuncture and herbal medicine.

- **Bowen therapy**: Uses a remedial body technique that is gentle and relaxing, helping the body's own healing resources to achieve balance and harmony which can help to relieve pain and discomfort.

- **Chinese herbal medicine**: Part of traditional Chinese medicine in which herbs are prescribed to restore balance to the opposing forces of energy (Yin/Yang).

- **Chiropractic therapy**: Focuses on the readjustment of the spine which practitioners believe to be the focus of disease.

- **Healing (therapeutic touch)**: Linked with the laying on of hands by Jesus Christ, and thus associated with Christianity. People with strong 'life energy' are able to transmit it to others by the laying on of hands.

- **Herbal medicine**: Plants and herbs used to treat disease and enhance well-being.

- **Homeopathy**: Used to mimic the symptoms of the disease in order to promote the body's own natural defenses and promote its ability to heal itself.

- **Iridology**: The iris is read and abnormal signs recorded. Uses diet, rest, exercise and fasting. Originates from Germany.

- **Kinesiology**: Biofeedback (muscle testing) is used to look at imbalances within the body that may cause diseases. Muscles are linked to internal organs, so muscle changes relate to diseases of particular organs.

- **Macrobiotics**: Eating provides a fundamental basic link to the environment. A link between Yin, Yang, Qi and food.

- **Massage**: Used for centuries by many different cultures to treat a range of disorders.

- **Meditation**: Focuses the attention on some subject to achieve calmness and relaxation. Can result in long-term health benefits.

- **Naturopathy**: Uses diet, massage and herbal medicine to encourage the body to heal itself. Many of the concepts underpinning this approach, including diet and exercise, have been adopted by traditional medicine.

- **Osteopathy**: Practitioners believe that the body cannot heal itself if the musculoskeletal system is misaligned. Therefore, they work on soft tissue (muscles and ligaments) to relieve pain, improve joint mobility and enhance general well-being.

- **Qi-gong**: Referred to as Chinese yoga, it includes meditation, breathing and movement, similar to t'ai chi.

- **Reflexology**: A method of diagnosis and treatment of conditions using pressure applied to the foot.

- **Reiki**: Practitioners remove energy blockages from the body by channelling energy through their hands into the patient.

- **Shiatsu**: Sometimes called acupressure, this technique from Japan involves applying pressure to specific points in the body such as P6 Nei Quan which is used for nausea.

- **T'ai chi**: Gentle exercise and movement designed to exercise the body and clear the mind for health and well-being. Originates from ancient China.

- **Yoga**: An ancient Indian philosophy which includes exercise and meditation designed as a path to spiritual enlightenment. Benefits include increased fitness and lower levels of stress and anxiety.

Further information can be found in many places on the Internet – see web sites at he end of the chapter.

CAM and pain

Many CAM therapies are often used for the relief of pain and anxiety (Astin, 1998). Pain clinics often recognize that such approaches can be beneficial to patients who are experiencing chronic pain. Thus approaches such as massage, healing, reflexology, acupressure, acupuncture and t'ai chi have all been used in this setting. As long as there is good communication between the therapist and the health-care practitioner, this should not be problematic.

The US Center for Complementary and Alternative Medicine (*nccam.nci.nih. gov*) classifies CAM into five main groups:

- biologically based
- alternative medical systems
- mind–body interventions
- manipulative and body-based methods
- energy therapies (Table 10.1).

Research by Dunn, Sleep and Collett (1995) explored the use of massage and aromatherapy in a group of 122 patients in an intensive care setting. Although the authors were unable to produce any statistical evidence of reduction in psychological stress indicators, or the patient's observed or reported ability to cope, the patients who received aromatherapy/massage reported a significantly greater

Table 10.1 Types of CAM therapies

Type	Element	Treatment
Biologically based	Dietary supplements, herbal, aromatherapy	Migraine, rheumatic pain, osteoarthritis
Alternative medical systems	Homeopathic, naturopathic, ayurveda, acupuncture	Knee pain, chronic headache
Mind–body	CBT, meditation, prayer, mental healing	Low back pain
Manipulation	Chiropractic, osteopathy, manipulation, massage	Low back pain
Energy	Energy fields, Qi-gong, reiki, therapeutic touch, pulsed magnetic therapy	Low back pain

improvement in mood and perceived levels of anxiety immediately following therapy. Because such self-reports cannot be considered objective, the researchers acknowledged that these findings could not therefore be generalized. Despite the lack of empirical evidence, however, the changes reported by the patients were considered to be important for the study. In relation to chronic pain, both anxiety and mood are considered to be important factors within the experience and as such a strategy which may improve these factors and consequently impact upon the pain is worth further consideration. Furthermore, the patient's comments on feeling better are significant for the chronic pain group, as this reinforces the issue of feeling in control and more positive about oneself.

An earlier study by Fraser and Ross Kerr (1993) looked at the effects of back massage on 21 elderly residents. Although the investigators in this study could not find any statistical evidence to support the use of such a strategy with their client group, again the verbal reports were very positive, in that the strategy improved communication and aided relaxation. The sample in this study was very small and there was a great variation in the medication intake and diagnosis for the patients, which could explain the lack of statistical evidence. However, consistent with the Dunn, Sleep and Collett (1995) study, Fraser and Ross Kerr (1993) highlight the positive effects of such approaches in making the patients 'feel better', which is an important issue for anyone with chronic pain.

Many articles advocate the use of aromatherapy for the treatment of painful conditions such as dysmenorrhoea, rheumatism and arthritis (Earle, 1994), but they are largely based on anecdotal evidence. The benefits of aromatherapy are highlighted by Price (1987, 1993), but these claims are supported by case studies rather than controlled research. However, the physiological basis on which the potential success of such an approach is well documented and is due to the close proximity of the receptors on the skin for touch (Aβ) and nociception (C fibres) (Melzack and Wall, 1991). There is, therefore, great potential for this strategy to be explored further as a nursing approach.

Touch

One aspect consistent in all of the reviewed studies on the use of massage is the concept of touch, the most basic of all of the primary senses; from birth to death, humans need to be touched. Doerhing (1989) suggested that a caring touch lasting just one second has the power to make individuals feel better. If anxiety is considered a pain amplifier, the reassurance associated with touch can reduce anxiety and so reduce pain. Nursing has the advantage of being in more direct contact with the patient than any other health-care profession, and consequently has the most potential to make a major contribution to care by utilizing the skill of touch.

The concept of touch can be simple, in that the touch of a hand can offer reassurance, caring, security and feelings of positive self worth (Carter, 1995). Alternatively, touch can be more complex, as described in the work of Krieger (1975) and Jurgens, Meehan and Wilson (1987) who advocate the use of therapeutic touch. There is some controversy associated with the use of therapeutic touch and some confusion between this term and the 'laying on of hands' (Jurgens, Meehan and Wilson, 1987) which sometimes appear to be used interchangeably. The original study by Krieger (1975) which explored the concept of therapeutic touch demonstrated an increase in haemoglobin values. However, this study was marred by methodological problems: the subjects were not defined and they were selectively assigned into treatment groups knowing which treatment they were receiving. The later study by Krieger (1975) was anecdotal and suggested that therapeutic touch could potentiate the relaxation response. It subsequently prompted further quasi-experimental studies. Heidt (1981) reported a significant decrease in anxiety amongst a group of cardiovascular patients receiving therapeutic touch compared to those receiving casual touch or verbal instruction, and these results were replicated in a study by Quinn (1982). In contrast, Randolph (1984) found no significant differences in physiological indicators of stress in a group of healthy college students.

These studies are all confounded by methodological problems: for example, Heidt (1981) carried out the treatment herself, Randolph (1984) used healthy subjects and her operational definition of therapeutic touch was significantly different from that of the others. Clearly, there is a need to support the concept of therapeutic touch beyond the placebo response with empirical evidence. However, humans do have a need to be touched, throughout life, to indicate love, reassurance and even joy. Although there may be no conclusive scientific evidence to support the therapeutic value of touch as a therapy, it is a fundamental means of communication and part of human nature and nursing care (Holden, 1991).

Music therapy

There has been much research into this approach. An early study by Altschuler (1948) highlighted that the use of music can potentially change an individual's mood, either consciously or subconsciously. The physiological rationale is based on the involvement of the thalamus as a relay station for emotions and feelings. This belief resulted in the development of the **Iso principle**, whereby music was matched and subsequently used to change a patient's mood. Later studies by Livingston (1979) evaluated music for prenatal classes, labour and delivery, and from his work he suggested that music therapy provided an excellent strategy for patients experiencing sensory restriction. He linked this with the sensory restriction work and highlighted how such experiences may precipitate boredom and anxiety. Furthermore, the author suggested that sensory deprivation can potentially result in the reticular activating system within the brain becoming overloaded with internal sensory experiences. Livingston (1979) went on to suggest that music therapy can counter the effects of sensory restriction by providing the reticular activating system with a pleasing, comforting or familiar level of stimulation.

Later research into music therapy has tended to explore two fields: music as a distraction therapy or the use of music to provide analgesia. The latter was based on the belief that music can stimulate the release of endorphins (Goldstein, 1980). A study by Updike (1990) explored the distraction therapy concept with the use of music for patients nursed in an intensive care setting. For the study 20 patients were recruited; the age range of the sample was 20–60 years. A choice of music was provided (classical or contemporary) and data were collected to measure response, along with interview notes before and after the music therapy. The findings of the study indicated a significant decrease in systolic blood pressure and a shift from anxiety and sadness to relaxation and calm, although the author did not indicate the source of these results. Updike (1990) also demonstrated a diminished pain experience in the sample.

Another study by Heitz, Symreng and Scamman (1992) examined the effects of music on pain, haemodynamic variables and respiration in a sample of 60 patients in a post-anaesthetic recovery room (PACU). For the study three groups of patients were selected; control (no music), control (headphones, no music) and experimental (headphones with music). The investigators found little significant difference in any of the measures between any of the groups. However, the music group were able to wait significantly longer before requiring any analgesia, and they recalled a significantly more pleasant recollection of their stay in the unit at one day and one month. The investigators cited other studies within the discussion and used them to compare results. For example, Taylor *et al.* (1998) investigated the effects of music therapy on a group of hysterectomy patients, on the first and second days after surgery. In this study the investigators demonstrated a significantly higher pain threshold in the experimental group, a finding which was further reinforced by Locsin (1981) who highlighted the reduced consumption of analgesia in the experimental group. The numbers in the studies were rather small, with a source of bias associated with the gender of the samples.

Melzack and Wall (1991) identified the potential pain-relieving properties of music in relation to the gate control theory, in that music can act as a distraction which closes the pain gate via central control.

Other studies in this field reinforce this proposal. For example, Wolfe (1978) investigated the use of music as part of a multidisciplinary pain programme for patients experiencing chronic pain. The music was used in conjunction with exercises and for leisure and relaxation. The results were presented in the form of two case studies, which highlighted the enjoyment of the music sessions, and the comments made by the patients reflected the benefits of using music in conjunction with exercise, supporting the potential distraction properties.

A study by Gardner, Licklider and Weisz (1960) demonstrated the effective use of music as a pain suppressant in over 5000 dental procedures, and a controlled study by Melzack, Weisz and Sprague (1963) demonstrated that music could totally abolish pain.

A major contributor in the field of music therapy is Deforia Lane (1992). As a registered nurse and director of music therapy, she further offers a possible explanation for the pain-relieving properties of music:

- Auditory stimulation occupies some of the neurologic pathways within the brain, thus resulting in fewer neurotransmitters being available to transmit the pain messages.
- Music can evoke intense emotions which stimulate the release of endorphins and hormones.
- Music has the power to reduce muscle tension which can intensify pain.
- Music may potentially reduce the feelings of helplessness and allow the individual to regain some control.

The studies reviewed into the use of music therapy remain inconclusive in their findings, but they appear to support the proposals of Lane (1992). Work into the use of music therapy is ongoing and it is considered, certainly in the USA, to be a very useful strategy. The types of environments which are considered most relaxing usually provide music in the background. Although, we should remember that an important element of music is self selection as some music can be annoying to some people.

There is no doubt that although the pain-relieving properties may be inconclusive, there is potential for using music just to make an experience more enjoyable or even relaxing. In addition, it provides a form of distraction, a theory on which all of the investigators agree. However, from a more cautious perspective the potential for music to evoke strong emotions needs consideration, as there is a need for staff to be able to deal with such emotions if they occur. Also, music can be individual; tastes are very variable, and a choice of music that is pleasant for one person may be actively unpleasant for another.

Distraction

It seems natural to assume that focusing attention away from the pain would be an appropriate strategy to cope with the pain. However, some early studies have demonstrated that this technique is not always effective.

For example, Leventhal *et al.* (1981, unpublished) found that women in childbirth found distraction ineffective. Similarly, McCaul and Haugvedt (1982) reported that although 80% of the subjects in their experimental study preferred to be distracted from their pain, in the cold pressor test they actually reported less pain with an 'attending to sensation' technique.

A review of studies into the use of distraction strategies was carried out by McCaul and Mallott (1984). They reviewed 17 studies in total between 1965 and 1980 that used cold pressor and other similarly painful stimuli. They concluded that distraction may provide a useful strategy to help with mild pain, but may become ineffective as the pain becomes more severe. Furthermore, McCaul and Mallott (1984) went on to develop a framework that may predict the effectiveness of the distraction technique. Within the framework two factors were identified as being indicators of potential success or failure of the technique: the interpretation of the pain experience, and the attentional capacity of the technique being used.

CAM and older adults

Older adults are more likely to experience at least one disease that is accompanied by chronic pain (Morris and Goli, 1994) as a consequence of the physiological changes that occur as a result of ageing. A community survey suggests that a high proportion of older adults experience persistent pain (Crook, Rivera L. and Browne, 1984) and a more recent survey suggests that this proportion can be as high as 50% of community-dwelling adults and 45–80% of nursing-home residents (Ferrell, 1991); 51% of nursing-home residents are reported to have pain on a daily basis (Ferrell, Ferrell and Osterweil, 1990).

Advances in pain management have identified a variety of pharmacological and non-pharmacological treatment options. However, studies describing pain management approaches for older adults are limited (Ferrell, 1991). Multimodal methods of pain control are claimed to be the most effective in this group, as the high risk of adverse effects from drug treatments complicates management (Forman and Stratton, 1991; Harkins and Price, 1992). Thus CAM may be appropriate as an adjuvant to traditional methods for older adults.

Review of the research

A systematic review of the literature dealing with this area revealed the following results.

Cognitive-behavioural therapy (CBT)/biofeedback

Psychological approaches for the management of pain have been developed and refined extensively since the introduction of the gate control theory of pain (Melzack and Wall, 1991), in particular for the management of chronic pain in adults. One such approach is based on the belief that by changing the individuals' thoughts and beliefs about their pain, they can adopt more positive coping strategies and subsequently regain control and consequently cope with ongoing pain. Many pain clinics around the world have adopted these approaches and report success in using CBT as a pain management strategy (Turk, Meichenbaum and Genest, 1983). It is believed that older adults do not respond well to CBT, and so in the literature they have either not been included in studies investigating CBT or they have been included within larger samples of younger adults, and so the effects specific to this group have not been identified. A wide range of psychological approaches have subsequently been developed and evaluated, but none of them have been explored with the older population.

One research study conducted in Canada recruited 28 elderly nursing-home residents and assigned them into two groups. The programme was conducted over a period of 10 weeks and included teaching the residents a range of skills including education, reconceptualization, relaxation, imagery, diversion and cognitive restructuring. The results of the study support the findings of others who demonstrate positive effects of psychologically based interventions, and the author concluded that CBT can be applied to nursing-home residents, but there is a need to be flexible to their needs and the group approach may not always be appropriate. He suggests that although it can be time consuming for staff, it is an approach that care staff could apply and has the potential to save care costs in terms of medication intake and nursing care related to pain.

More recently, Kerns, Otis and Marcus (2001) report a case study of a 72-year-old man referred to a pain centre and offered the opportunity to take part in CBT. This study further supports the positive findings suggested by Cook (1995) and suggested that CBT is well suited to the treatment of older people with chronic pain.

Finally, 22 nursing-home residents were invited to participate in a study by Strine (2002) in which they were randomly assigned to a biofeedback or waiting list group and subsequently monitored for 10 weeks. The results of the study indicate that biofeedback has potential efficacy for pain reduction among older people resident in nursing homes. When viewed collectively, the studies appear to suggest the potential effectiveness of psychologically based programmes for older people in care homes, provided resource issues and training can be addressed.

Massage

The earliest paper in this group presents the findings of a one-year project investigating the effects of gentle massage in two groups of elderly nursing-home residents suffering from chronic pain and dementia in New York. The study was facilitated by a qualified massage therapist, and 59 of 71 residents completed the 12-week programme (Sansone and Schmitt, 2000). Dementia and/or pain was identified using the Minimum Data Set (MDS) assessment, and then the resident's carer and/or family member was invited to take part in the training of 'tender touch'. Data were collected on pain and anxiety/agitation during the 3-month study period. The nursing assistants commented that they used the strategy when walking residents, and it helped to calm them down.

Family members also made positive comments. The paper contains some really moving accounts of family experiences. In conclusion, the authors found that the carers enjoyed using the approach, and pain and anxiety scores fell during the study period. Although this approach could be perceived as time consuming, the study found that after 1–2 hours of training the staff/carers could provide tender touch during periods of feeding or moving residents, and so it could potentially be incorporated into mainstream care tasks rather than being an 'extra'.

Another paper that examined the effects of aromatherapy/massage is that of Kunstler, Greenblatt and Moreno (2004). They highlighted how in 1998 the American Geriatric Society issued guidelines for the management of pain in the elderly, in which they recommended both pharmacological and non-pharmacological management of pain. They used a multiple single-subject design within an 816-bed long-term care facility. Four residents were recruited into the study and the data collected included pain assessment and observations/comments from the residents. Residents included in the study had to score >24 on the Mini-Mental State Examination (MMSE) and to be able to sign the consent form. The sessions were conducted by a certified therapeutic recreation specialist (CTRS) and consisted of a 30-minute hand massage and aromatherapy session in the early evening three times per week for 12 weeks. The authors reported the case studies and were able to demonstrate statistically significant reductions in participants' pain perceptions during intervention and also improved sleep patterns (although sample size small). Interestingly, part of the intervention within this study incorporated efforts to create a more positive environment in which relaxation could take place; this is similar to the findings of the author's own work (Schofield, 1996, 2002a,b; Schofield and Davis, 1998a,b, 2000).

Relaxation

McBee, Westreich and Likourezos (2004) conducted a study in nursing homes in the USA to investigate the effects of a 10-week programme of relaxation training. Fourteen residents participated in the study and were given a once-weekly session which covered the principles of relaxation along with the various different approaches which included meditation, music therapy, aromatherapy, and yoga and poetry readings. Group members were interviewed before and after the sessions about life satisfaction and their experiences of pain. After the interventions the group reported feeling 'less sad' and experienced less pain, although this was not significantly significant. Although the numbers in the study were very small, again this approach did not cause any harm and positive comments from the residents themselves indicate that this is an approach worthy of further investigation.

Exercise

A different perspective is adopted in the study by Simmons et al. (2002) who investigated the impact of exercise on pain. This study involved randomization of residents into a control group who received no treatment and the experimental group who participated in a 32-week exercise/endurance programme. The programme consisted of mobility training and stand-ups. Data were collected using the Geriatric Pain Measure and average mobility was measured before and after intervention. No significant changes in pain were observed with either group during the study, but the mobility of the experimental group improved over time. However, the investigators concluded that this intervention was ineffective over time; furthermore it would appear to be rather labour-intensive in terms of the staff commitment necessary to conduct the exercises 2-hourly for 32 weeks.

Qi therapy

A further study in this section involved a randomized controlled trial investigating the effects of Qi therapy in a group of older people in Korea (Tse, Pun and Benzie, 2005). The principles behind the approach are based on the Chinese philosophy of the vital energy (Qi) that flows through the body which can be restored through medical Qi-gong, which is similar to the laying on of hands or healing philosophies. For this study 43 participants from a residential care community were randomly assigned into a control (general care) or Qi therapy group. Pain and mood was assessed before intervention and weekly after intervention for 6 weeks. The results suggest that Qi therapy significantly reduced pain and improved mood in the experimental group. This was a small study with some promising results. However, further work would need to carried out and issues regarding the employment of a Qi master would need to be conducted, as well as wider issues regarding each of the complementary therapy studies and psychological interventions that have been reviewed appears to be related to the issue of control. Control is generally perceived as a valuable strategy for coping with pain.

T'ai chi

T'ai chi chuan means 'supreme ultimate boxing' (Sandlund and Norlander, 2000). It originated in China about 300 years ago and is based on the Taoist philosophy of Yin and Yang or opposing forces combined with breathing techniques. Today t'ai chi is widely practised around the world as a method of relaxation and moderate exercise. It is noted for its flowing, slow, dance-like movements and its function as a system of callisthenics and self-defence, as well as being a vehicle for meditation and spiritual well-being. The dynamics of t'ai chi emphasize movement in graceful patterns, deep diaphragmatic breathing, simple weight shifts moving from deep relaxation to full speed and force with balance and whole body connection. The art of t'ai chi has five basic principals: relaxation, separating Yin and Yang, turning the waist, keeping the back erect and total body movement.

Advocates of t'ai chi report many benefits including relief from muscular tension, reduced anxiety, stress and pain and increased balance, self-awareness and strength. It has been suggested that t'ai chi provides a defence against arthritis, malfunctioning metabolism and many other illnesses. Two reasons are proposed as a rational for this:

- Participants have to be very focused to gain inner peacefulness, thus excluding other distractions and stressors.
- The smooth slow rhythmic movements promote muscular relaxation and flexibility.

However, there is very little scientific evidence to support the use of t'ai chi and its potential positive impact, although there is evidence to support the use of yoga (Roberts, 1973), relaxation (Everly and Rosenfield, 1981), exercise (Griest *et al.*, 1979) and martial arts (Konzak and Boudreau, 1984), all of which may contribute to the positive effect of t'ai chi, either individually or in combination.

Research

As nursing strives to become a profession, it is a requirement that practice is underpinned by sound theoretical evidence. Furthermore, health care is increasingly under pressure to be underpinned by evidence. Therefore, research must be used to support approaches, albeit qualitative research that emphasizes the quality-of-life issues which are often impacted by complementary approaches. In order for nurses to take on board these approaches, several key issues must be addressed: research, professional, clinical and educational.

Professional

The Nursing and Midwifery Council (NMC) requires that nurses are accountable for their own practice, and it is also a requirement that nurses ensure that they have the appropriate education and training. The Bolam test can be used in a court of law to determine whether or not the practitioner practised within the guidelines of recommended practitioners. Therefore, a nurse practising acupuncture, for example, will be judged against a qualified acupuncturist. This also raises important insurance issues.

Clinical

Time and resources are always at a premium within nursing practice. In order to practice many of the complementary approaches, it is necessary to spend considerable time creating the right sort of environment. This is not always appropriate in busy wards where all sorts of events are occurring.

Educational

Courses in the various complementary therapies vary greatly. For example, acupuncture can be studied during a short 3 day course or alternatively a 3 year programme, so careful selection of educational programmes is required. Furthermore, as mentioned previously, the NMC requires that the nurse ensures he/she has the appropriate training.

Conclusion

The 20th century brought medicine into the scientific age. Advances in medicine, the introduction of technological approaches and new pharmacological discoveries have moved medicine away from the concept of holism – the approach that highlights the relationship between the spiritual, physical and environmental aspects. Nevertheless, it must not be forgotten that drug catastrophes such as thalidomide have highlighted that modern medicine cannot always deliver, and in some cases can actually cause harm.

Modern medicine is often considered to be cold and inhuman, even uncaring. Patients and practitioners have become increasingly disillusioned with it, and are turning towards complementary approaches which offer a role for them as part of their own management.

Nursing models also emphasize holistic care, so nurses are in an ideal position to promote and in some cases practice complementary therapies, as they fit well with the holistic philosophy of nursing. However, complementary approaches still require empirical evidence to support their use and legislation to ensure that they are monitored closely. Further empirical evidence is required to protect patients and ensure that they have access to the best possible care.

References

Altschuler J. (1948) A psychiatrist's experience with music as a therapeutic agent, in *Music and Medicine*, (eds S. Schullian and H. Schoer), Schuman, New York.Astin, J.A. (1998) Why patients use alternative medicine – results of a national study. *JAMA* **279**(19), 1548–53.

Carter, B. (1995) Complementary therapies and management of chronic pain. *Paediatric Nursing*, **7**(3), 18–22.

Cook, A. (1995) *Cognitive-behavioural pain management for elderly nursing home residents*. Doctoral Thesis, University of Manitoba.

Crook, J., Rivera L. and Browne, G. (1984) The prevalence of pain complaints among a general population. *Pain*, **18**, 299–314.

DH (1993) *Report on the Taskforce on the Strategy for Research in Nursing, Midwifery and Health Visiting*. Department of Health, London.

Department of Health (2000) *Complementary Medicine: Information Pack for Primary Care Groups*. HMSO, London.

Doerhing, K.M. (1989) Relieving pain through touch. *Advancing Clinical Care*, Sept/Oct, 32–3.

Dunn, C., Sleep, J. and Collett, D. (1995) Sensing an improvement: an experimental study to evaluate the use of aromatherapy, massage and periods of rest in an intensive care unit. *Journal of Advanced Nursing*, **21**, 34–40.

Earle, L. (1994) *Vital Oils*. Vermillion, London.

Ernst, E., Resch, K.L., Mills, S., Hill, R., Mitchell, A. and Willoughby, M. *et al.* (1995) Complementary therapies – a definition. *British Journal of General Practice*, **45**, 506.

Everly, G.S. and Rosenfield, R. (1981) *The Nature and Treatment of the Stress Response*. Plenum Press, New York.

Ferrell, B.A., Ferrell, B.R. and Osterweil, D. (1990) Pain in the nursing home. *Journal of the American Geriatric Society*, **90**, 409–14.

Ferrell, B.R. (1991) Pain management in elderly people. *Journal of American Geriatrics Society*, **39**, 64–73.

Forman, W. and Stratton, M. (1991) Current approaches to chronic pain in older patients. *Geriatrics*, **46**, 47–52.

Fraser, J. and Ross Kerr, J. (1993) Psychological effects of back massage on elderly institiutionalized patients. *Journal of Advanced Nursing*, **18**, 238–45.

Gardner, W.J., Licklider, J.C.R. and Weisz, A.Z. (1960) Suppression of pain by sound. *Science*, 132, 32–3.

Goldstein, A. (1980) Thrills response to music and other stimuli. *Physiological Psychology*, **8**(1), 126–9.

Griest, J.H., Klein, M.H., Eischens, R.R., Faris, J., Gurman, A.S. and Morgan, W.P. (1979) *Exercise and Mental Health. The Series in Health Psychology and Behavioural Medicine*. Hemisphere Publishing, Washington, DC.

Harkins, S.W. and Price, D.D. (1992) Assessment of pain in the elderly, in *Handbook of Pain Assessment* (eds D.C. Turk and R. Melzack). Guilford Press, New York.

Heidt, P. (1981) Effect of therapeutic touch on anxiety levels of hospitalized patients. *Nursing Research*, **30**(1), 32–7.

Heitz, L., Symreng, T. and Scamman, F. (1992) Effect of music therapy in the postanesthesia care unit. A nursing intervention. *Journal of Anaesthesia Nursing*, **7**(1), 22–31.

Holden, R.J. (1991) An analysis of caring: attributions, contributions and resolutions. *Journal of Advanced Nursing*, **16**, 893–8.

Howell, J. (1993) Complementary medicine. BMA pushes for more research. [comment]. *BMJ*, **307**(6904), 625.

Jurgens, A., Meehan, T. and Wilson, H. (1987) Therapeutic touch as a nursing intervention. *Holistic Nursing Practice*, **2**(1), 1–13.

Konzak, B. and Boudreau, F. (1984) *Canada's Mental Health*. December, 2–7.

Krieger, D. (1975) Therapeutic touch: the imprimatur of nursing. *American Journal of nursing*, **75**(5), 784–87.

Kunstler R., Greenblatt, F. and Moreno, N. (2004) Aromatherapy and hand massage: therapeutic recreation interventions for pain management. *Therapeutic Recreation Journal*, **38**(2), 133–46.

Lane, D. (1992) Music therapy: a gift beyond measure. *Oncology Nursing Forum*, **19**(6), 863–7.

Leventhal, H., Shacham, S., Boothe, L. and Leventhal, E. (1981) *The role of attention in distress and control during childbirth.* Unpublished MPhil studies, Wisconsin.

Livingston, M. (1979) Music for the childbearing family. *Nursing,* **8**, 363–7.

Locsin, R. (1981) The effects of music on pain in selected postoperative patients. *Journal of Advanced Nursing,* **6**, 19–25.

Kerns R., Otis J.D. and Marcus, K.S. (2001) Cognitive-behavioural therapy for chronic pain in the elderly. *Clinics in Geriatric Medicine,* **17**(3), 503–23.

McBee, L., Westreich, L. and Likourezos, A. (2004) A psychoeducational relaxation group for pain and stress management in the nursing home. *Journal of Social Work in Long Term Care,* **3**(1), 15–28.

McCaul, K. and Haugvedt, C. (1982) Attention, distraction and cold pressor pain. *Journal of Personality,* **48**, 494–504.

McCaul, K. and Mallott, J.M. (1984) Distraction and coping with pain. *Psychological Bulletin,* **95**(3), 516–33.

Melzack, R. and Wall, P.D. (1991) *The Challenge of Pain.* Penguin, London.

Melzack, R., Weisz, A.Z. and Sprague, L.T. (1963) Strategems for controlling pain: contributions of auditory stimulation and suggestion. *Experimental Neurology,* **8**, 239–47.

Montbriand, M. (1993) Freedom of choice: an issue concerning alternative therapies chosen by patients with cancer. *Oncology Nursing Forum,* **20**(8), 1195–201.

Morris, C.E. and Goli, V. (1994) The physiology and biomedical aspects of chronic pain in later life, in *Older Women with Chronic Pain* (ed. K.A. Roberto), 9–24. Haworth Press, New York.

Murray, J. and Shepherd, S. (1988) Alternative or additional medicine? A new dilemma for the doctor. *Journal of the Royal College of General Practitioners,* **38**, 511–14.

Nursing & Midwifery Council (2004) *NMC Code of Professional Conduct: Standards for Conduct Performance and Ethics.* NMC, London.

Price, S. (1987) *Practical Aromatherapy.* Thorsons, London.

Price, S. (1993) *Aromatherapy Workbook.* Thorsons, London.

Quinn, J. (1982) *An investigation of the effects of therapeutic touch done without physical contact on the state anxiety of hospitalized patients.* PhD dissertation, New York University.

Randolph, G. (1984) Therapeutic and physical touch: physiological response to stressful stimuli. *Nursing Research,* **33**(1), 33–6.

Roberts, N. (1973) *The Yoga Thing.* Hawthorne Books, New York.

Sandlund, E.S. and Norlander, T. (2000) The effects of Tai Chi Chuan relaxation and exercise on stress responses and well being: an overview of the research. *International Journal of Stress Management,* **7**(2),139–49.

Sansone, P. and Schmitt, L. (2000) Providing tender touch massage to elderly nursing home residents: a demonstration project. *Geriatric Nursing,* **21**(6), 303–8.

Schofield, P.A. (1996) Snoezelen: its potential for people with chronic pain. *Journal of Complementary Therapies in Nursing and Midwifery*, **2**(1), 9–12.

Schofield, P.A. (2002a) Snoezelen: an alternative environment for relaxation in the management of chronic pain. *British Journal of Nursing*, **11**(12), 811–19.

Schofield, P.A. (2002b) The feasibility of using Snoezelen within palliative care. *International Journal of Palliative Nursing*, **93**, 124–30.

Schofield, P.A. and Davis, B. (1998a) Sensory deprivation: the concept as applied to chronic pain. *International Journal of Disability and Rehabilitation*. **20**(10), 357–66.

Schofield, P.A. and Davis, B. (1998b) Snoezelen and chronic pain: developing a study to evaluate its use (Part 1) *Journal of Complementary Therapies in Nursing and Midwifery*, **4**, 66–72.

Schofield, P.A. and Davis, B. (2000) Sensory stimulation (Snoezelen) versus relaxation for the management of chronic pain. *International Journal of Disability and Rehabilitation*, **22**(15), 675–82.

Simmons, S.F., Ferrell, B.A. and Schnelle, J.F. (2002) Effects of a controlled exercise trial on pain in nursing home residents. *Clinical Journal of Pain*, **18**, 380–5.

Strine, G.N. (2002) *Self-reports of pain reduction through paced respiration and heart rate variability biofeedback with nursing home residents*. Doctoral Thesis, Widener University, MA.

Taylor, L.K., Kuttler, K.L., Parks, T.A. and Milton, D. (1998) The effect of music in the postanesthesia care unit on pain levels in women who have had abdominal hysterectomies. *Journal of PeriAnesthesia Nursing*, **13**(2), 88–94.

Ter Riet, G., de Craan, A.T.M., de Boer, A. and Kessels, A.G.H. (1998) Is placebo analgesia mediated by endogenous opioids? A systematic review. *Pain*, **76**, 273–5.

Tse, M.M.Y., Pun, S.P.Y. and Benzie, I.F.F. (2005) Pain relief strategies used by older people with chronic pain: an exploratory survey for planning patient-centred interventions. *Journal of Clinical Nursing*, **14**, 315–20.

Turk, D., Meichenbaum, D. and Genest, M. (1983) *Pain and Behavioural Medicine*. Guilford Press, New York.

Updike, P. (1990) Music therapy results for ICU patients. *Applied Research*, **19**(1), 39–45.

Wolfe, D. (1978) Pain rehabilitation and music therapy. *Journal of music therapy*, **XV**(4), 162–78.

Web sites

Better Health Channel (Victoria, Australia): <*http://www.betterhealth.vic.gov.au/bhcv2/ bhcarticles.nsf/pages/tr_complementarytherapies?open*>

Cochrane Collaboration: <*http://www.cochrane.org*>

Department of Health (UK): <*http://www.dh.gov.uk/PolicyAndGuidance/ HealthAndSocialCareTopics/ComplementaryAndAlternativeMedicine/fs/en*>

Expert Committee on Complementary Medicines in the Health System (Australia): <*http://www.tga.gov.au/docs/html/cmreport.htm*>

National Center for Complementary and Alternative Medicine (USA): <*http://nccam. nih.gov*>

National Library for Health (NHS searchable database of national and international resources): <*http://www.library.nhs.uk/Default.aspx*>

Wikipedia article: <*http://en.wikipedia.org/wiki/Complementary_medicine*>

Function and rehabilitation

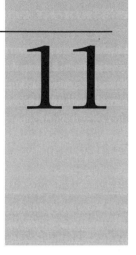

Denis Martin

The aim of this chapter is to discuss the concept of function and rehabilitation in the management of pain in older people. In particular, there is a specific focus on physiotherapy rehabilitation to maintain and restore function.

The importance of function

A central component of pain management for older people, as well as for all other populations, is the promotion of function. Many drugs and medicines are currently available and in widespread use that can help older people with pain, but that approach is often insufficient on its own: there ais a range of other, non-pharmacological, approaches to managing pain that can be employed in parallel, to help people live their lives to their full capacity (Ahmad and Goucke, 2002; Gibson, 2006). Many of these non-pharmacological approaches involve approaches including physiotherapy that come into the category of rehabilitation – the restoration or improvement of function (Stucki, Ewert and Cieza, 2002).

Function should be considered in a wide sense to include such diverse activities as standing for long periods of time, walking for a set distance or time, doing everyday housework chores, getting dressed in the morning, work, sexual activity and participation in different community activities. For people who have difficulty in coping with pain, all of these activities and more can be affected, to the detriment of their quality of life (Scudds and Robertson, 2000; Reyes-Gibby, Aday and Cleeland, 2002; Thomas *et al.*, 2004). For older people (and others) who are having problems coping with pain, the impact of pain on function can be limited by rehabilitation – regaining as normal a pattern of work and social life that can be achieved (DoH, 2006).

The International Classification of Function, Disability and Health

Function has a very significant position in modern thinking about health and well-being. This is seen by the importance given to the World Health Organization's International Classification of Function, Disability and Health (ICF) (WHO, 2001). The activities that are listed above are items included in the WHODAS II questionnaire, which was developed from the ICF and is used to measure disability and function in people with health conditions (Von Korff *et al.*, 2005). The ICF provides a clear description of the different components of function and how they relate to each other. As well as being a very useful theoretical classification system, it provides a practically useful framework for explaining, understanding, planning, implementing and evaluating rehabilitation strategies.

In the ICF health is described in terms of function. When health is regarded as being positive this is described as functioning and when health is regarded as being compromised or negatively affected this described as **dysfunctioning** or **disability**.

Within the ICF **function** has two components: body structure and body functions; and activity and participation.

- **Body structures** are anatomical entities such as muscles, nerves and bones. In terms of pain and its impact they include structures involved in movement and the nervous system. Body functions include both physiological and psychological mechanisms. From the perspective of pain and its impact these include sensory and nociceptive functions, mental functions and functions that are related to movement.
- The term **activity** is used within the ICF to describe the capacity of a person to carry out a task or an action. Here **capacity** refers to what he or she **can do**. **Participation** relates to the person's performance or taking part in social situations. It is a reference to what he or she **actually does**.

Using the above terms, the ICF discusses three levels of dysfunctioning or disability:

- When there are problems with body structures and body functions these are described as **impairments**.
- When someone has a reduced ability to carry out a task or action – problems with capacity – these are referred to as **activity limitations**.
- Finally, problems with performance or taking part in social situations are described as **participation restrictions**.

The ICF also emphasizes **context** in function and disability. Context includes personal factors ranging from age and sex to life experience, health experience and ways of coping with problems. Also included in context are environmental factors such as social support and attitudes of friends, families and social contacts; social and health policies; and technology. (In the ICF the concept of a standard environment is used when describing a person's performance, a concept that has generated some debate (Nordenfelt, 2003).)

The value of the ICF can be seen by comparing it to the previous system from which it evolved. Under that system – the International Classification of Impairments, Disabilities and Handicaps (ICIDH) – health and disability were treated as two distinctly separate concepts. In the ICF, however, they are linked together as different presentations of function. In contrast to the ICF, the ICIDH was interpreted as lending very little, if any, real importance to the influence of environmental factors. Within the ICIDH, health problems were described as a disease or disorder that developed in a step-by-step way, beginning with impairment, progressing to disability and then developing into handicap. The ICF differs from the ICIDH in that it expands that concept to allow for independence and more fluid relationships between impairment, activity limitations and participation restrictions. As such, it is more compatible with a biopsychosocial model of health that is currently seen to be of value in the management of people with chronic pain (Main and Spanswick, 2000; Keefe *et al.*, 2004).

The biopsychosocial model of pain management

Managing pain based on the biopsychosocial model recognizes that pain can have physiological, psychological and environmental effects, and that physiological, psychological and environmental factors can influence the impact of pain (Hanson and Gerber, 1989; Main and Spanswick, 2000). The biopsychosocial model has become popular in the field of the management of long-term conditions in general and in chronic pain in particular.

Chronic pain

Chronic pain is a long-term condition in its own right and a common co-morbidity of other long-term conditions (Von Korff *et al.*, 2005). It is an example of a lived-in long-term condition – a condition for which a cure has yet to be found (Christianson, Taylor and Knutson, 1998). Until now, with examples of initiatives to change systems, health care has been driven by systems and approaches that have been designed to deal with conditions for which there is an obtainable cure. However, these systems and approaches do not meet the needs of people with a long-term condition like chronic pain.

The overarching problem is that these systems and approaches are based on a biomedical model of disease and cure. Within a biomedical model pain is seen to be a sensation that comes about following damage to tissues – a symptom of an underlying injury or disease. This way of thinking may be of some use in consideration of acute pain (though not always), but it is too simplistic to accurately represent the complex, multidimensional phenomenon that is chronic pain. For example, the biomedical model does not adequately address the emotional aspects of pain and it requires pain to be linked with actual tissue damage, neither of which is in line with current research evidence and accepted expert opinion. In contrast, the wider perspective offered by the relationships among physiological, psychological and environmental factors in the biopsychosocial model is in line with current definitions of pain such as: 'an unpleasant sensory and emotional experience associated with actual or potential tissue damage, or described in terms of such damage' (Merskey and Bogduk, 1994). Because of this, the biopsychosocial model has provided the basis for developing more comprehensive approaches to managing chronic pain than those that are purely pharmacological and medical(Keefe et al., 2004).

Biopsychosocial approaches to managing pain place a particular focus on facilitating the person with chronic pain to live as full a life as possible through improving their capacity to carry out tasks and actions, and by encouraging the person to take part in social activities. There is, therefore, a clear link between the ICF and biopsychosocial approaches to rehabilitation in managing pain (Soukup and Vollestad, 2001; Steiner et al., 2002; Chwastiak and Von Korff, 2003).

Age-related aspects of pain

It seems to be commonly believed that pain is a greater problem for older people than for their younger counterparts. Such a view is likely to involve an underestimation of the problem of pain in people who do not fall into the category of 'older', as well as involving a lack of understanding of the quality and quantity of evidence about age-related effects on pain and its impact. Currently, evidence suggests that, in general, within the overall population, pain is indeed more common in older people than in younger ones (Harkins, 2001; Smith, 2001; Helme and Gibson, 2001; Thomas et al., 2004). That picture, though, is complicated by findings that the age-related prevalence of pain may level out or decline when it comes to people aged over 70 years (Helme and Gibson, 2001). Even that finding is difficult to interpret, because the lower prevalence may be more precisely described as a lower prevalence of people reporting pain: the lower reported figure may be due to problems in communicating the presence of pain, or stoicism, rather than simply meaning that pain is not present. There is also some evidence to suggest that changes in neurophysiological structures and function with increased age may lead to a decrease in the perception of pain (Gibson *et al.*, 1994). This picture is complicated by the possibility that the methods used in studies that derive such conclusions may not rule out alternative reasons for their findings. In addition, many aspects of this field have not been thoroughly investigated and thus there remain many gaps in the knowledge base. Also, much remains to be uncovered about how psychosocial and environmental factors interact with pain in older people. These include attitudes and beliefs about pain, health co-morbidities, loss of social support networks and bereavement (Helme and Gibson, 2001).

Most importantly, however, from the perspective of function and rehabilita-tion, the evidence strongly suggests that for those older people who are vulnerable to the disabling effects of chronic pain, those disabling effects are likely to be greater than in their younger counterparts (Mobily *et al.*, 1994; Helme and Gibson, 2001; Thomas *et al.*, 2004). As Thomas *et al.* (2004) put it: 'the experience of pain becomes more disabling with age'. Not surprisingly in such a complex area, however, some research does not agree with that stance (Jakobsson, Hallberg and Westergren, 2003), indicating that this is still a live area for further investigation to clarify the position. It is useful at this stage, when grey areas of evidence are being outlined, to make the point that because the effects of ageing on health and well-being are not completely predictable, and because the impact of pain is not uniform, it is not valid to view older people or older people with pain as a homo-geneous group (Gibson, 2006). A simple illustration of this is the experience of retirement. For some older people retirement is a time to take things easy and relax, while for others the reality of retirement is a struggle against low income and poor housing (Burke, 2006). A relatively simple environmental difference like that may have profound health effects.

Because difficulties in coping with pain can reduce function, an older person with pain living in the community is at risk of avoidable hospital admission or admission to long-term care. Similarly, for an older person already in care who is having difficulty in coping with pain, there is a risk that their optimal independent function will be further reduced. This reflects a common feature of the impact of pain – a cycle of disuse and inactivity. This cycle in turn leads to a further reduction in function through decreases in strength, mobility and fitness and accompanying psychological effects such as focusing on pain, decreased confidence in abilities, fear of causing harm and worsening mood. What is required to break the cycle is the restoration of function, or at least the deceleration of its decline when the overall health of the person is in decline. Hence, there is a clear role for rehabilitation to reduce activity limitation and participation restriction in older people who are having difficulty coping with pain (Thomas *et al.*, 2004).

The role of physiotherapy in rehabilitation

Physiotherapy has a central rehabilitation role to play in helping people, including older people, to manage pain. The British Pain Society (see web site at end of chapter) outlines a range of core components of pain management programmes, and it is interesting to note that most of these are applicable to physiotherapy. For example, physiotherapy methods can help the person to increase strength, mobility and fitness. They can also help to improve people's confidence in their ability to perform activities and tasks. Physiotherapy methods can also incorporate relaxation techniques, the provision of relevant information and education, and guidance, feedback and support during a person's gradual return to activities of daily living. Similarly, the Department of Health's Musculoskeletal Services Framework (DH 2006) outlines the role of pain management services that include roles of relevance to physiotherapy and rehabilitation: providing people with information about their pain; providing guidance in practical ways of remaining active despite the presence of pain; increasing function and helping to reduce distress and unwarranted fears about what it means for the person to be in pain.

This is an expansion of the more traditional role of physiotherapy, which involved the application of techniques to people who primarily acted as passive patients, within a biomedical model of treatment. As discussed above, the biomedical model is too narrow to meet the needs of people with chronic pain: the expansion of the physiotherapy role represents the evolution of practice within a biopsychosocial model with a focus on improving function that has been affected by pain, rather than only focusing on attempting to correct putative causes of pain (Harding and Williams, 1995; Jones and Martin, 2003). In this context physiotherapy aims not only to reduce pain where possible but also to help people develop skills to deal with the disabling effects of pain.

The role of CBT

Cognitive-behavioural principles can be adapted into physiotherapy and rehabilitation for people with chronic pain (Harding and Williams, 1995; Moseley, 2002; Johnstone, Donaghy and Martin, 2003). Cognitive-behavioural therapy (CBT) has gained an important place in pain management within a biopsychosocial model. In pain management the basis of CBT is that the impact of pain on people is connected to the attitudes and beliefs that people have about their pain (Stroud *et al.*, 2000). People with chronic pain often report that they have recurring thoughts such as 'what have I done to deserve this?' or 'I can't take the pain any more', and negative emotions like anger, frustration and low mood.

Such negative thinking and emotion is perfectly normal given the presence of long-term pain, but it can lead to unhelpful behaviours like withdrawing from social contact and inactivity – participation restriction and activity limitation – which only add to the problems of the person with chronic pain (Keefe *et al.*, 2004). CBT aims to help people with chronic pain to become aware of the problems associated with their negative thoughts and feelings; it helps people to challenge their negative thoughts and develop positive ways of behaving (Williams *et al.*, 1993; Morley, Eccleston and Williams, 1999).

Giving people information about pain and helping them to understand how it can affect their life is an important part of rehabilitation. It can help to address misplaced beliefs about pain that can interfere with function and it can help people to develop self management strategies (Burton *et al.*, 1999; Butler and Moseley, 2003; Moseley, 2004).

Exercise

Exercise is one of the main physical therapies that can promote function in people with chronic pain, including older people. Among the benefits are improved strength, mobility and fitness; improved mood; and potentially some degree of reduction in pain. Where overall health is in decline, exercise can be used to slow down the rate of that decline.

Research suggests that the important thing is to exercise, regardless of the form that it takes (Liddle, Baxter and Gracey, 2004). This is important because there are many different types of exercise – some well established, some in vogue and some that have become less fashionable. When considering the type of exercise, factors such as individual preference, individual lifestyle, belief in benefits and health status should be considered (CSP, 2006). Supervision of the exercise and provision of useful feedback is also important (Liddle, Baxter and Gracey, 2004). Exercise should have an overall aim of improving activity and participation. Within this context exercise can include everyday activities like housework and social activities like dancing.

It is not sufficient just to recommend exercise, as there are barriers that can prevent people with chronic pain from following that advice. People with low back pain, for example, may have a misplaced fear of movement causing damage that can prevent them from exercising (Vlaeyen and Linton, 2000). A common problem encountered in helping people with chronic pain to improve activity and participation levels is a tendency to try to do too much on 'good' days and then do nothing on 'bad' days. This overactivity/underactivity cycle is likely to lead to a decrease in function over time. The complementary techniques of pacing and goal setting are useful ways of levelling out these excessive peaks and troughs of overactivity and underactivity (Fey and Fordyce, 1983; Harding and Williams, 1995).

Pacing and goal setting

Pacing is a simple idea about developing a pattern of activity and participation that is characterized by small periods of activity punctuated with regular breaks from that activity (Nielson, Jensen and Hill, 2001). In order to do this, the person needs to calculate what are known as **activity tolerances**. Tolerances are quantifiable measures, usually time or distance, of an activity that brings on increases of pain and/or fatigue. An example is standing tolerance – the time a person can stand in one place before pain and/or fatigue increases. Having determined the tolerance for the activity, the person sets a baseline for that activity. The baseline is a reduced quantity of activity below tolerance level (often 50–80% of the tolerance level). Pacing then involves interrupting the activity when the baseline has been reached, and resuming after a period of rest or alternative activity. Although it is a simple idea, working out tolerances and baselines can be quite complex and the physiotherapist has an important role in offering guidance, feedback and support in this.

Goal setting involves clearly defining what the person intends to do and then setting out a series of targets, the successful completion of which will lead to the achievement of the goal. Like pacing it is a simple idea in theory but often quite complex to put into practice and the person will benefit from guidance, feedback and support from the physiotherapist. The SMART principle should be applied in goal setting. This means that each goal should be *s*pecific, *m*easurable, *a*ctivity related, *r*ealistic and *t*ime related:

- **Specific** means that the goal should be clearly defined. A goal such as wanting to dance at a wedding can be more clearly defined as wanting to dance for ten minutes with the groom's father at your daughter's wedding.

- **Measurable** means that the person can clearly recognize that the goal has been achieved.

- **Activity-related** means that the achievement of the goal means that the person has to actively do something.

- **Realistic** means that the achievement of the goal is a realistic possibility under the control of the person's efforts. There are many factors outwith the person's control, such as lack of time or money, that can prevent the achievement of a goal.

- **Time-related** means that a date or end point is established by which time the person will be expected to have achieved the set goal.

Although, like pacing, it is a relatively simple idea, goal setting can be challenging. The physiotherapist can work with the person to improve activity and participation by offering guidance, feedback and support on goal setting and, within that, prioritizing, delegating and planning tasks.

Pain flare-ups

Flare-ups of pain, when the pain reaches an unusually high level, can be a difficult barrier to improving or maintaining levels of function. Common physical triggers that can cause pain levels to flare up include:

- staying put in a particular position or posture for too long;
- taking part in a certain activity for too long;
- excessive effort, such as trying to lift a very heavy weight.

Emotional stress can also cause pain to flare up. A role for physical therapists is to offer guidance about how to decrease the frequency of flare-ups of pain, and make flare-up more manageable when it happens.

One way of dealing with flare-ups of pain is to reduce their frequency by helping the person to identify the triggers and thus avoid the activities that tend to bring them on. Another way is to help the person to develop a plan to use a range of methods of dealing with the flare-up when it happens. Physiotherapy methods such as relaxation, pacing and goal setting, heat, cold, transcutaneous electrical nerve stimulation (TENS) and stretching can be used at this time. Other flare-up management techniques that people can include in their plan can include stress reduction, dealing with negative thoughts, improving communication with others, overcoming sleep disturbances, distraction, viewing pictures, visualization and listening to music.

The therapist's knowledge, attitudes and beliefs

Factors that are perhaps less obvious in the successful rehabilitation of the person with pain are the knowledge, attitudes and beliefs of the health professional about chronic pain and the person with chronic pain (Jones and Martin, 2003). The situation regarding knowledge, attitudes and beliefs is probably best described as variable (Jones and Martin, 2003). Problems arise when the physiotherapist (or other professional) has a predominantly biomedical view of pain, which can lead to a mismatch between the needs of the person and the physiotherapy and rehabilitation methods offered (Blomqvist, 2003).

As mentioned in the introduction, the discussion of function and rehabilitation for the person with chronic pain has had a particular focus on physiotherapy. It is important to note that best practice should aim for interdisciplinary working with colleagues from occupational therapy, psychology, medicine, nursing, pharmacy and support groups (Wagner, 2000) while still acknowledging the value of different professional perspectives (Jones and Martin, 2003).

Conclusion

Older people with pain are vulnerable to its disabling effects, and physiotherapy has an important role to play in providing rehabilitation to counter this. Throughout the text reference has been made to the idea of offering guidance, feedback and support to help the person to manage their pain. This reflects a personal view that the physiotherapist's role has many features of coaching. It requires an understanding of the specific needs of the person. It involves them as active participants in their own management, working together to agree goals and explaining why activity and participation is both possible and worth achieving. It is also worth noting that much of the information informing the discussion of rehabilitation and pain management for older people is based on research and practice that is either not age specific or exclusively for people described as 'younger'. For example, research studies that provide evidence to inform practice often include an upper age limit in the 60s in their inclusion criteria. In the absence of age-specific information it can be argued that using such evidence and expert opinion to inform practice for older people has validity (Sorkin *et al.*, 1990; Gibson *et al.*, 1994) and it is up to physiotherapists to adapt these approaches to individual circumstances to best meet the needs of the older person with chronic pain (Lansbury, 2000; Barry *et al.*, 2003).

References

Ahmad, M. and Goucke, C.R. (2002) Management strategies for the treatment of neuropathic pain in the elderly. *Drugs Aging*, **19**(12), 929–45.

Barry, L.C., Guo, Z., Kerns, R.D., Duong, B.D., Reid, M.C. and Funotuinal, A. (2003) Self-efficacy and pain-related disability among older veterans with chronic pain in a primary care setting. *Pain*, **104**, 131–7.

Blomqvist, K. (2003) Older people in persistent pain: nursing and paramedical staff perceptions and pain management. *Journal of Advanced Nursing*, **41**(6), 575–84.

Burke, E.J. (2006) Psychosocial factors in pain management of the older patient, in *Clinical Management of the Elderly Patient in Pain*. (eds G. McCleane and H. Smith), pp. 219–37. Haworth Medical Press, New York.

Burton, A., Waddell, G., Tillotson, K.M. and Summerton, N. (1999) Information and advice to patients with back pain can have a positive effect. A randomized controlled trial of a novel educational booklet in primary care. *Spine*, **24**(23), 2484–91.

Butler, D. and Moseley, G.L. (2003) *Explain Pain*. NOI Group Publishing, Adelaide.

CSP (2006) *Clinical Guidelines for the Physiotherapy Management of Persistent Low Back Pain. Part 1 Exercise*. Chartered Society of Physiotherapy, London.

Christianson, J.B., Taylor, R. and Knutson, D. (1998) *Restructuring Chronic Illness Management: Best Practices and Innovations In Team-Based Treatment*. Jossey-Bass, San Francisco.

Chwastiak, L.A. and Von Korff, M. (2003) Disability in depression and back pain: evaluation of the World Health Organization Disability Assessment Schedule (WHO DAS II) in a primary care setting. *Journal of Clinical Epidemiology*, **56**(6), 507–14.

DH (2006) *Musculoskeletal Services Framework*. Department of Health, London.

Fey, S.G. and Fordyce, W.E. (1983) Behavioral rehabilitation of the chronic pain patient. *Annual Review of Rehabilitation*, **3**, 32–63.

Gibson, S.J. (2006) Older people's pain. International association for the study of pain. *Clinical Updates*, **14**(3), 1–4.

Gibson, S.J., Katz, B., Corran, T.M., Farrell, M.J. and Helme, R.D. (1994) Pain in older persons. *Disability and Rehabilitation*, **16**, 127–39.

Hanson, R.W. and Gerber, K.E. (1989) *Coping with Chronic Pain: A Guide to Patient Self-management*. Guilford Press, New York.

Harding, V. and Williams, A.C.deC. (1995) Extending physiotherapy skills using a psychological approach: cognitive-behavioural management of chronic pain. *Physiotherapy*, **81**(11), 681–8.

Harkins, S.W. (2001) Aging and pain, in *Bonica's Management of Pain*, 3 edn. (ed. J.D. Loeser), pp. 813–23. Lippincott, Williams & Wilkins, Philadelphia.

Helme, R.D. and Gibson, S.J. (2001) The epidemiology of pain in elderly people. *Clinics in Geriatric Medicine*, **17**, 417–31.

Jakobsson, U., Hallberg, R.H. and Westergren, A. (2003) Pain management in elderly persons who require assistance with activities of daily living: a comparison of those living at home with those in special accommodation. *European Journal of Pain*, **8**, 335–44.

Johnstone, R., Donaghy, M. and Martin, D.J. (2003) A pilot study of a cognitive-behavioural therapy approach to physiotherapy, for acute low back pain patients, who show signs of developing chronic pain. *Advances in Physiotherapy*, **2**, 182–8.

Jones, D. and Martin, D.J. (2003) Chronic pain, in *Interventions for Mental Health: An Evidence Based Approach for Physiotherapists and Occupational Therapists* (eds T. Everett, M. Donaghy and S. Feaver), pp. 136–45. Butterworth-Heinemann, Edinburgh.

Keefe, F.J., Rumble, M.E., Scipio, C.D., Giordano, L.A. and Perri, L.M. (2004) Psychological aspects of persistent pain: current state of the science. *Journal of Pain*, **5**(4), 195–211.

Lansbury, G. (2000) Chronic pain management: a qualitative study of elderly people's preferred coping strategies and barriers to management. *Disability and Rehabilitation*, **22**, 2–14.

Liddle, S.D., Baxter, G.D. and Gracey, J.H. (2004) Exercise and chronic low back pain: what works? *Pain*, **107**(1–2), 176–90.

Main, C.J. and Spanswick, C.C. (2000) *Pain Management: An Interdisciplinary Approach*. Elsevier Health Sciences, London.

Merskey, H. and Bogduk, N. (1994) *Classification of Chronic Pain*. IASP Press, Seattle.

Mobily, P.R., Kerr, H.A., Wallace, R. and Chung, Y. (1994) An epidemiological analysis of pain in the elderly: the Iowa 65-plus Rural Health Study. *Journal of Aging and Health*, **6**, 139–54.

Morley, S., Eccleston, C. and Williams, A.C.deC. (1999) Systematic review and meta-analysis of randomised controlled trials of cognitive behaviour therapy for chronic pain in adults, excluding headache. *Pain*, **80**(1–2), 1–13.

Moseley, G.L. (2002) Physiotherapy is effective for chronic low back pain. A randomised controlled trial. *Australian Journal of Physiotherapy*, **48**, 297–302.

Moseley, G.L. (2004) Evidence for a direct relationship between cognitive and physical change during an education intervention in people with chronic low back pain. *European Journal of Pain*, **8**(1), 39–45.

Nielson, W.R., Jensen, M.P. and Hill, M.L. (2001) An activity pacing scale for the chronic pain coping inventory: development in a sample of patients with fibromyalgia syndrome. *Pain*, **89**(2–3), 111–5.

Nordenfelt, L. (2003) Action theory, disability and ICF. *Disability and Rehabilitation*, **25**(18), 1075–9.

Reyes-Gibby, C.C., Aday, L. and Cleeland, C. (2002) Impact of pain on self-rated health in the community-dwelling older adults. *Pain*, **95**(1–2), 75–82.

Scudds, R.J. and Robertson, J.M. (2000) Pain factors associated with physical disability in a sample of community-dwelling senior citizens. *Journal of Gerontology. Series A, Biological Sciences and Medical Sciences*, **55**(7), M393–9.

Smith, B. (2001) Chronic pain: a challenge for primary care. *British Journal of General Practice*, **51**, 524–6.

Sorkin, B.A., Rudy, T.E., Hanlon, R.B., Turk, D.C. and Steig, R.L. (1990) Chronic pain in old and young patients: differences appear less important than similarities. *Journal of Gerontology*, **45**(2), 64–8.

Soukup, M.G. and Vollestad, N.K. (2001) Classification of problems, clinical findings and treatment goals in patients with low back pain using the ICIDH-2 beta-2. *Disability and Rehabilitation*, **23**(11), 462–73.

Steiner, W.A., Ryser, L., Huber, E., Uebelhart, D., Aeschlimann, A. and Stucki, G. (2002) Use of the ICF model as a clinical problem-solving tool in physical therapy and rehabilitation medicine. *Physical Therapy*, **82**(11), 1098–107.

Stroud, M.W., Thorn, B.E., Jensen, M.P. and Boothby, J.L. (2000) The relation between pain beliefs, negative thoughts, and psychosocial functioning in chronic pain patients. *Pain*, **84**(2–3), 347–52.

Stucki, G., Ewert, T. and Cieza, A. (2002) Value and application of the ICF in rehabilitation medicine. *Disability and Rehabilitation*, **24**(17), 932–8.

Thomas, E., Peat, G., Harris, H., Wilkie, R. and Croft, P.R. (2004) The prevalence of pain and pain interference in a general population of older adults: cross-sectional findings from the North Staffordshire Osteoarthritis Project (NorStOP). *Pain*, **110**, 361–8.

Vlaeyen, J.W.S. and Linton, S.J. (2000) Fear-avoidance and its consequences in chronic musculoskeletal pain: a state of the art. *Pain*, **85**, 317–32.

Von Korff, M., Crane, P., Lane, M., Miglioretti, D.L., Simon, G., Saunders, K., Stang, P., Brandenburg, N. and Kessler, R. (2005) Chronic spinal pain and physical–mental comorbidity in the United States: results from the national comorbidity survey replication. *Pain*, **113**(3), 331–9.

WHO (2001) *International Classification of Functioning, Disability and Health: ICF.* World Health Organization, Geneva.

Wagner, E.H. (2000) The role of patient care teams in chronic disease management. *British Medical Journal*, **320**, 569–72.

Williams, A.C.deC., Nicholas, M.K., Richardson, P.H., Pither, C.E., Justins, D.M., Chamberlain, J.H., Harding, V.R., Ralphs, J.A., Jones, S.C., Dieudonne, I., Featherstone, J.D., Hodgson, D.R., Ridout, K.L. and Shannon, E.M. (1993) Evaluation of a cognitive behavioural programme for rehabilitating patients with pain. *British Journal of General Practice*, **43**, 513–8.

Web sites

British Pain Society (a multidisciplinary professional organization): <*www.britishpainsociety.org*>

Department of Health, Musculoskeletal Services Framework: <*http://www.library.nhs.uk/musculoskeletal/ViewResource.aspx?resID=148887*>

Future directions

12

Pat Schofield

Introduction

Where do we go from here? What needs to be done to improve practice in the future? What contribution can be made by all members of the multidisciplinary team to improve pain management? How can the team work together with the older person to address the inadequacies that currently exist? And how can the team include the older person as part of this process? These are all questions that will be discussed in this chapter under four main headings: clinical, research, education and professional aspects.

Clinical aspects

Geriatric medicine developed out of necessity, which sets it apart from other medical specialities that evolved from the development of a unique body of knowledge. Similarly, the speciality of pain and ageing remains in its infancy. The disparities that exist in age-related pain management have been highlighted by many in emergency care, outpatient settings and long-term care facilities, to name but a few. It is widely recognized that the problems exist in many disciplines (Haley, 1983; Brown *et al.*, 2003; Neighbor, Honnor and Kohn, 2004; Won *et al.*, 2004).

It has now been acknowledged that older adults in pain are not a chronologically older version of younger pain patients (Weiner, 2006). One of the first difficulties that we encounter when working with older adults is the definition of 'old', which may vary according to culture or context. For example 'old' may relate to retirement, length of time lived or becoming a grandparent. There are many definitions, and some flexibility is required; for example, people under 75 may be dealt with by geriatricians but it is more likely that people over 75 will require specialist geriatric care, as they are more likely to be frail. A third group is described as the oldest, sickest and most frail group with the most complicated medical problems (Hazzard *et al.*, 1994). However, Nelson Mandela, at 88 years old, embodies accumulated knowledge, wisdom, depth of experience and resilience (Gibson, 2006).

The world's population is ageing. It is anticipated that by 2050 the proportion of people over 65 will rise from 17.5% to 36.3%, and the over-80 group will more than triple (US Bureau of the Census, 2004). Even more worrying is the fact that the number of gerontological nurses available to care for this population is already inadequate (Hollinger-Smith, 2003).

The dichotomy with chronic pain in older adults is that this group actually appear to have a lower burden of psychosocial disruption and less of a desire to take medications, with a greater belief in self-management than their younger counterparts (Weiner *et al.*, 2006). However, as we know, there is more likelihood that the older population will be more likely to have co-morbidities and associated polypharmacy, along with an increased risk of social isolation, limited income and decreased neurological and physical function (Edwards, 2005). Furthermore, evidence suggests alterations in pain processing and perceptions of pain (Gagliese and Farrell, 2005). But of course we must not assume that pain is an inevitable part of ageing. As discussed in Chapter 1, this belief can result in barriers to effective pain management (Figure 12.1).

Many older adults can manage the pain themselves, with limited or no help from health professionals. But where this does not occur, a number of compre-

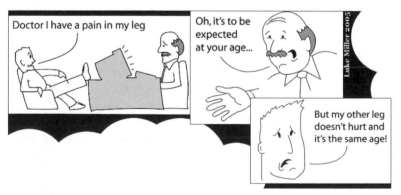

Figure 12.1   So is pain inevitable? (copyright Luke Miller, 2005)

hensive guidelines are available. The American Geriatrics Society and the Australian Pain Society have produced guidelines for residential care (see web sites at end of chapter), and the British Pain Society will soon be publishing guidelines for the assessment of pain in older adults.

The key principals in managing pain in older adults that have been highlighted within the recent guidelines includes the following:

- Pharmacological therapy for persistent pain is most effective when combined with non-pharmacological approaches.
- The choice of analgesic drugs for older people requires an understanding of age-related pharmacokinetic and pharmacodynamic changes and must consider the impact of co-morbid disease and concurrent medication use.
- Simple analgesics are most appropriate for mild to moderate pain.
- NSAIDs and cyclooxygenase-2 inhibitors should be used with caution.
- Benefit/risks should be balanced with all drugs.
- Non-pharmacological treatments which have some evidence base include:
  - graded exercise
  - heat/cold
  - TENS
  - relaxation
  - cognitive-behavioural therapy
  - educational programmes
  - social support programmes
  - some complementary therapies
  - acupuncture
  - joint injections and surgery
  - multidisciplinary management.

The evidence for intrathecal pumps and spinal cord stimulators is still inconclusive (Gibson, 2006). In terms of home-based care, some attempts have been made to apply multidisciplinary management programmes in the community and some evidence recommends the use of multimodal management within care home settings. Figure 12.2 shows a care pathway that has been developed for the management of pain in care homes (Schofield and Reid, 2006).

Research aspects

Although over 4000 research papers are published annually relating to pain, less than 1% of them focus on the needs of older adults. The are two ways of looking at this disparity. First, should we be treating older adults any differently from their

Could this resident be in pain?

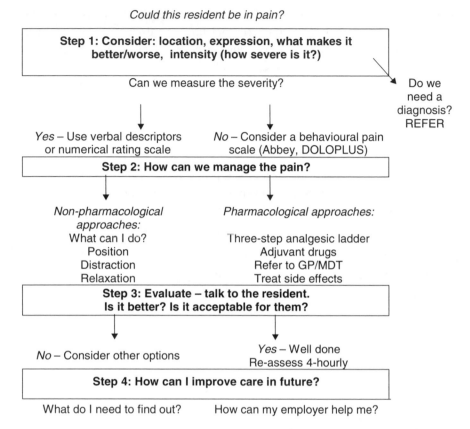

Step 1: Consider: location, expression, what makes it better/worse, intensity (how severe is it?)

Can we measure the severity?

Do we need a diagnosis? REFER

Yes – Use verbal descriptors or numerical rating scale

No – Consider a behavioural pain scale (Abbey, DOLOPLUS)

Step 2: How can we manage the pain?

Non-pharmacological approaches:
What can I do?
Position
Distraction
Relaxation

Pharmacological approaches:

Three-step analgesic ladder
Adjuvant drugs
Refer to GP/MDT
Treat side effects

Step 3: Evaluate – talk to the resident. Is it better? Is it acceptable for them?

No – Consider other options

Yes – Well done
Re-assess 4-hourly

Step 4: How can I improve care in future?

What do I need to find out?   How can my employer help me?

Figure 12.2   Care pathway for care-home residents (Schofield and Reid, 2006)

younger counterparts? It could be argued that by focusing research specifically upon their needs we are in danger of segregating them. The alternative perspective suggests that older adults are unique and different in their experiences and needs from their younger counterparts, and therefore these needs should be highlighted. Of course some also suggest that gerontology is not high-tech or glamorous, and health-care professionals therefore are not attracted to this field. Furthermore, research into this group can be challenging, with issues around consent, concordance and dementia which can cause problems for the researcher.

Geriatric medicine is a highly specialized area, as management of older people requires a very different perspective from dealing with younger patients. The spectrum of complaints, manifestations of distress and differential diagnosis is very different. Functional status is more important and recovery less dramatic. Although many of the problems associated with ageing cannot be cured, much can be done to improve discomfort and disability which constitutes the 'art' of geriatric care (Ferrell, 1996). Therefore, geriatric pain management could be considered an art in which much can be achieved. The high risk associated with pharmacological management in this group leaves the potential for creative and innovative management that can impact upon quality of life, social care and self-management – all of which are worthy areas of investigation.

There is a move in the UK to promote research into pain management for older people. Already, there is evidence to underpin effective pain assessment practice and several researchers have looked at the pain experiences of the care home population (Schofield, 2006) and made recommendations for the educational requirements of staff (Allcock, McGarry and Elkan, 2002). Research in this field lends itself well to qualitative paradigms that explore the experiences of older adults, but there is also room for quantitative methodologies that explore different interventions.

So, as Gibson (2002) said 'it is time to grasp the nettle' and focus on the development of good-quality research studies that raise the profile of pain in older adults, demonstrate effective methods of pain assessment and promote the most appropriate methods of management.

Educational aspects

A recent study by Lovheim et al. (2006) highlighted that in a sample of 3724 residents, 56.7% were experiencing pain. From those in pain, 27.9% were receiving no analgesia or regular medication for their pain. The authors also demonstrated that for 72.7% of these residents, the staff member who claimed that they knew the resident the best thought that they were actually receiving the best treatment for the pain, when in fact they were not receiving any at all (Ferrell, 1991; Melding, 1991; Gibson, 2002; Cohen-Mansfield, 2004). This is not a new finding; many investigators have previously identified the poor management of older people in pain. But it is the most recent study, and demonstrates that things have not improved at all in the last 10–15 years.

The only way that this situation can improve is to develop better communication between older people and their carers, and this can only happen if the carers understand the experiences of the older people in their care. Issues around pain assessment and management can be addressed. Many pain assessment tools have been developed that are appropriate for measuring pain in older adults, from simple numerical scales to the more complex measures such as the Abbey or DOLOPLUS scales (see Chapter 4). Information regarding management in this group is available, and there is scope for further research on complementary therapies which can be used to complement the traditional pharmacological approaches and reduce the need for high doses of drugs. Such creativity can only occur if the staff have the right level of understanding of pain in older adults.

So education is the key. A number of small studies have demonstrated the potential for education of staff to improve pain management, and make recommendations for developments in this area (Ferrell, Ferrell and Rivera, 1995; Ross and Crook, 1998; Blomqvist and Edberg, 2002). All levels of staff need to understand older adults' pain experience, which will enable them to recognize pain and be creative and innovative in their approach to care. Many advances have been made since the introduction of the gate control theory in terms of understanding and education, and this must continue to encompass the specific needs of older adults.

Professional aspects

This section should focus on the professional issues concerned with pain management. However, it is important to state at the outset that pain management is not the sole concern of any single profession. Throughout this book we have attempted to demonstrate the various aspects of pain management of older adults and the various contributions that can be made by all members of the multidisciplinary team. Since Melzack and Wall (1965) introduced their gate control theory of pain it has been acknowledged that just as pain is a multidimensional experience which impacts upon physical, psychological and social aspects of the individuals' life, in turn it can also be influenced by these aspects. As such treatment is not just about injections or drugs, but also includes psychological management or counselling.

Learning point

- What professional groups work within your clinical area?
- What contribution to pain management can be made by each of these members of the team?
- If you are unsure, make it your priority to find out.

Report on the European Week Against Pain (EWAP)

The World Health Organization warns that pain is a global social concern. In 2000 there were more than 60 000 000 people over 60 years old and this number will increase to a staggering 2 billion by the year 2050. Pain is the symptom most frequently reported by older people: on average, 73% of older people in a community say that they are experiencing pain. The evidence supports an age-related increase in pain prevalence.

In September 2006 a press conference was held to launch the start of the IASP Global Year Against Pain, focusing on pain in older persons, and EFIC's 6th European Week Against Pain (EWAP) had the same theme. Why is pain in older people important (IASP/EFIC, 2006)?

- Adults of advanced age form a larger proportion of the population in Europe than elsewhere in the world. In the near future, Europe's most important health problem will be pain in elderly people.

- Pain is a very common problem for elderly people. Chronic pain affects more than 50% of older people living in the community, and more than 90% of nursing-home residents. At a minimum, 50% of the older citizens of Europe suffer from chronic pain.

- Pain is a major health-care problem in Europe. The incidence of chronic disease is higher among older adults than in the rest of the population. Although acute pain may reasonably be considered a symptom of disease or injury, chronic and recurrent pain is a specific health-care problem, a disease in its own right.

- Elderly adults have reduced sensitivity to noxious stimuli, but when older persons do report pain, they are likely to be affected with greater levels of underlying pathology than younger individuals who report the same level of pain.

- Elderly adults commonly have age-associated psychosocial difficulties, such as retirement, loss of support from family and friends, bereavement, loss of independence and hospitalization. These factors constitute an added burden and may influence the expression of pain and its response to treatment.

- More than one clinical diagnosis typically contributes to chronic pain in older adults. Impaired quality of life secondary to pain may be expressed by depression, anxiety, sleep disruption, appetite disturbance and weight loss, cognitive impairment and limitations in the performance of daily activities.

- Cancer is the second leading cause of death for adults over 65 years of age, and 67% of all cancer deaths occur in those over age 65.

- More than a quarter (26%) of cancer patients aged over 65 years of age who are in daily pain did not receive any analgesia.

- The effective treatment of pain in adults of advanced age requires specialized knowledge and training in pain management. When formulating a treatment plan, one needs to be aware of the important influence of concurrent medications and the potential impact of co-morbid medical and psychosocial problems. Familiarity with important drug interactions that may affect analgesic actions, and may have side effects, is also important. Health-care workers need to be aware of relative and absolute contraindications to certain drugs that are commonly used by older adults.

The European Federation of IASP Chapters (EFIC) devised a European survey to gather information on various problems associated with 'pain in the elderly'. The objectives of this survey were to explore issues surrounding the day-to-day management of pain amongst older people and to explore general attitudes towards pain. These aims were explored from both a patient's and a health-care professional's perspective.

This survey took place in France, Germany, Italy, Poland and the United Kingdom. In each location 45 minute in-depth telephone interviews were conducted with general practitioners (GPs) (6), patients (6) and nurses (5). All patients were over 65 years old and had been suffering from chronic pain for at least 6 months. Health-care professionals (HCPs) consisted of GPs and nurses (district nurse/community nurse, nurse working in care home or residential home, or hospital nurse) who regularly see patients, or care for people in this age range. Key findings from the survey are:

- All key stakeholders need to be involved in setting the agenda for pain management in older people.
- Curricula need to address knowledge and attitudes around pain in this group.
- Funding bodies need to prioritize pain research into this group.
- Focus needs to be given to the educational needs of primary care practitioners.
- Access to multidisciplinary care should be provided for all older people.
- Pain medicine needs to be combined with geriatric medicine in order to provide expert care.
- Special attention should be given to pain for people in residential care, at the end of life and for those with cognitive or communication impairment.
- Pain is not a normal part of ageing.
- Training and resources in less developed countries must be improved.
- Cooperation of all health-care professionals, funding bodies, carers, patients and their relatives is paramount.

The EFIC/IASP survey and press release (see web sites listed at end of chapter) summarizes the important issues regarding pain management in the older population in a way that is succinct and represents the global perspective. This book has attempted to address some of the key areas that can be addressed by nurses and health-care staff working on the front line. Such contributions must not be undervalued. Scientists and epidemiologists may consolidate the evidence and make recommendations for best practice. But front-line care staff deal with older adults in pain on a day-to-day basis and as such they are in an unique position to understand the needs of their older patients, and improve assessment and management of pain. It is hoped that this book will help them to do so.

References

Allcock, N., McGarry, J. and Elkan, R. (2002) Management of pain in older people within a care home: a preliminary study. *Health and Social Care In the Community*, **10**(6), 464–71.

Blomqvist, K. and Edberg, A. (2002) Living with persistent pain: experiences of older people receiving home care. *Journal of Advanced Nursing*, **40**(3), 297–306.

Brown, J.C., Klein, E.J., Lewis, C.W., Johnston, B.D. and Cummings, P. (2003) Emergency department analgesia for fracture pain. *Annals of Emergency Medicine*, **42**(2), 197–205.

Cohen Mansfield, J (2004) The adequacy of the minimum data set: assessment of pain in cognitively impaired nursing home residents. *Journal of Pain and Symptom Management*, **27**(4), 343–51.

Edwards, R.R. (2005) Age-associated differences in pain perception and pain processing, in *Pain in Older Persons, Progress in Pain Research and Management Seattle* (eds D.K. Gibson and S.J. Weiner), pp. 45–65. IASP Press, WA.

Ferrell, B.A., Ferrell, B.R. and Rivera, L. (1995) Pain in cognitively impaired nursing home patients. *Journal of Pain and Symptom Management*, **10**, 591–8.

Ferrell, B.R. (1991) Pain management in elderly people. *Journal of American Geriatrics Society*, **39**, 64–73.

Ferrell, B.R. (1996) Non-drug interventions, in *Pain in the Elderly* (eds B.R. Ferrell and B.A. Ferrell), pp. 35–44. IASP Press, Seattle.

Gagliese, L. and Farrell, M. (2005) The neurobiology of ageing, nociception and pain processing, in *Pain in Older Persons, Progress in Pain Research and Management* (eds S. Gibson and D. Weiner), pp. 25–44. IASP Press, Seattle, WA.

Gibson, S. (2002) *Pain in Older Persons*. Presentation at the World Pain Congress. IASP, San Diego.

Gibson, S. (2006) Older people's pain. *Pain: Clinical Updates*, **XIV**, 3.

Haley, W.E. (1983) Priorities for behavioural intervention with nursing home residents: an exploration of prevalence, staff perspectives and practical aspects of measurement. *International Journal of Behavioural Geriatrics*, **1**, 47–51.

Hazzard, W.R., Bierman, E.L., Blass, J.P., Ettinger, W.H. and Halter, J.B. (1994) *Principals of Geriatric Medicine and Gerontology*. McGraw Hill, New York.

Hollinger-Smith, L. (2003) How to care for an aging nation: start with educating the educators. *Journal of Gerontological Nursing*, **29**(3), 23–7.

IASP/EFIC (2006) *Pain in Older Persons Media Pack*. International Association For the Study of Pain, European Federation of IASP Chapters, <*http://www.efic.org/pressrelease2006.pdf*>.

Lovheim, H., Karlsson, S.H., Sandman, P., Kallin, K. and Gustafson, Y. (2006) Poor staff awareness of analgesic treatment jeopardises adequate pain control in the care of older people. *Age and Ageing*, **35**(3), 257–61.

Melding, P.S. (1991) Is there such a thing as geriatric pain?: guest editorial. *Pain*, **46**, 119–21.

Melzack, R. and Wall, P.D. (1965) Pain mechanisms: a new theory. *Science*, **150**, 971.

Miller, L. (2005) Physiological and biochemical change, in *The Management of Pain in Older People – A Distance Learning Package* (eds P.A. Schofield, M. Dunham, C. Black and B. Aveyard), ISBN 1-902411-39-0, University of Sheffield.

Neighbor, M.L., Honnor, S. and Kohn, M.A. (2004) Factors affecting emergency department opioid administration to severely injured patients. *Academy of Emergency Medicine*, **11**(12), 1290–6.

Ross, M. and Crook, J. (1998) Elderly recipients of nursing home services: pain disability and functional competence. *Journal of Advanced Nursing*, **27**(6), 1117–26.

Schofield, P.A. (2006) Pain management of older people in care homes: a pilot study. *British Journal of Nursing*, **15**(9), 509–14.

Schofield, P.A. and Reid, D. (2006) The assessment and management of pain in older people: a systematic review of the Literature. *International Journal on Disability and Human Development*, **5**(1), 9–15.

US Bureau of the Census (2004) *We the People: Aging in the United States*. Census 2000 Special Reports CENSR-19, US Bureau of the Census, Washington, DC.

Weiner, D.K. (2006) Editorial: pain and ageing: a call to those with the power of inquiry, the skills to teach and the desire to heal. *Pain Medicine*, **7**(1), 57–9.

Weiner, D.K., Rudy, T.E., Morrow, L., Slaboda, J. and Leiber, S.J. (2006) The relationship between pain, neurophysical performance and physical function in community dwelling older adults with chronic low back pain. *Pain Medicine*, **7**, 60–70.

Won, A.B., Lapane, K.L., Vallow, S., Schein, J., Morris, J.N. and Lipitz, L.A. (2004) Persistent non-malignant pain and analgesic prescribing patterns in elderly nursing home residents. *Journal of the American Geriatric Society*, **52**(6), 867–74.

Web sites

American Geriatrics Society, *The Management of Persistent Pain in Older Persons*: <*http:// www.americangeriatrics.org/products/positionpapers/JGS5071.pdf*>

Australian Pain Society, *Pain in Residential Aged Care Facilities – Management Strategies*: <*http://www.apsoc.org.au/owner/files/9e2c2n.pdf*>

European Federation of IASP Chapters (EFIC): <*http://www.efic.org/index.html*>

Facts on Pain in Older Persons: <*http://www.efic.org/facts2006.pdf*>

International Association for the Study of Pain: <*http://www.iasp-pain.org*>

United Nations Department of Economic and Social Affairs, Population Division, *World Population Ageing: 1950–2050*: <*http://www.un.org/esa/population/ publications/worldageing19502050/*>

US Bureau of the Census, *We the People: Aging in the United States. Census 2000 Special Reports CEN3R-19*: <*http://www.census.gov/prod/2004pubs/censr-19.pdf*>

Index